Life, with Cancer

Life, with Cancer

The Lauren Terrazzano Story

Frank Terrazzano & Paul Lonardo

Foreword by Anna Quindlen

Health Communications, Inc.
Deerfield Beach, Florida

www.hcibooks.com

A portion of the proceeds from the sale of this book will be donated to Joan's Legacy: Uniting Against Lung Cancer, The Lung Cancer Alliance, and to fund scholarships through the Lauren Elizabeth Terrazzano Memorial Scholarship Fund at Columbia University's School of Journalism.

Library of Congress Cataloging-in-Publication Data

Terrazzano, Frank, author.
  Life, with cancer : the Lauren Terrazzano story / Frank Terrazzano, Paul Lonardo.
      pages cm
ISBN 978-0-7573-1663-0 (pbk.)
ISBN 0-7573-1663-8 (trade paper)
ISBN 978-0-7573-1664-7 (epub) (print)
1. Terazzano, Lauren, -2007—Health.   2. Lungs—Cancer—Patients—United States
  —Biography.   3. Journalists—United States—Biography.   I. Lonardo, Paul, author.
II. Title.
RC280.L8T47 2012
616.99'4240092—dc23
[B]

                                                                            2012023357

Publisher: Health Communications, Inc.
        3201 S.W. 15th Street
        Deerfield Beach, FL 33442-8190

Cover image ©Veronica Marino
Cover design by Dane Wesolko
Interior design by Lawna Patterson Oldfield
Interior formatting by Dawn Von Strolley Grove

Quod in vita facimus in aeternum resonat

"What we do in life echoes in eternity"

—Cicero

Contents

Acknowledgments

Losing a child to the dread disease of cancer is something you can never, ever prepare for as a parent. Lauren, our only child, was diagnosed with lung cancer at the age of thirty-six, and our world as we knew it came to an end.

We would have less than three more years together, and even that did not prepare her mom, Ginny, and me for the enormity of the grief we would experience when her courageous battle was lost.

Trying to come to terms with our loss inspired me to write this book about a beautiful young lady who believed that the "pen is mightier than the sword." Lauren chose to use her pen as a light to shine into dark places, exposing society's many shortcomings. Through her writing, Lauren championed the cause for abused children, the elderly, and the homeless in an attempt to make life better for all; she truly became a voice for the voiceless.

A most loving and caring daughter, her passing has left a void in our life that will never be filled. We desperately want to understand the reason that a beautiful, healthy, and talented young lady who was not a heavy smoker came to contract this scourge of a disease. Our

Lauren spent part of those final three years asking similar questions and raising public awareness about lung cancer.

The journey continues for my wife, Ginny, and me. However, we take much solace knowing that our Lauren's footprint will forever remain in the sands of time for all to see.

We love and miss her so very, very much.

In recognition of those who stood by Lauren during her illness and filled her life with so much joy, I would like to take this opportunity to express my sincerest gratitude by thanking five woman who I consider my daughter's de facto siblings for their kindness and the unwavering moral support they showed to her during her battle. Sylvia Adcock, Monica Quintanilla, Leah Ritchie, Tomoeh Murakami Tse, and Dina Fernandez were always there!

My thanks for the anecdotes from her many loving and caring journalism colleagues and to *Newsday* for permitting excerpts from Lauren's "Life, with Cancer" columns to be reprinted in this biography.

A heartfelt thank-you to Lauren's doctors and nurses for their kindness during the course of her treatment, with special thanks to Dr. Raja Flores, Dr. Akhtar Ashfaq, and Dr. Benvenisty for their unending support and advice to Lauren.

To Linda Konner for believing in this book and working with us when no other literary agent would. To editor Candace Johnson for her assistance in making this book better than I could ever have imagined.

To Anna Quindlen for all your kindness remembering Lauren and sharing your wonderful words!

Paul Lonardo, my coauthor, for were it not for his guidance and writing expertise, my dream and labor of love for this book about my beautiful daughter Lauren's travails would have languished and not have come to fruition.

Finally, my wife, Ginny, and I are grateful to all our friends for their wonderful support, with special thanks to good friends Patti and Larry Giangregorio, Barbara and Donald Greer, and their daughter Katie MacLeod, for constantly reaching out to us as Lauren waged her courageous battle.

—*Frank Terrazzano*

Foreword

Reporters are simply different from their civilian counterparts. We see things differently. Almost reflexively, we absorb images, details, impressions, and scribble them into our ever-present notebooks. It's not that we are any more observant by nature than other people. We just know that we have to pay attention in a particular way, for the sake of readers.

Lauren Terrazzano was a reporter her entire adult life, and, by anyone's account, a very good one. She was part of a team at Long Island's *Newsday* that won the Pulitzer Prize for spot news reporting, and she was one of those whom younger colleagues admired and tried to emulate.

She followed the path so many of us in the newspaper business have taken. In the beginning she covered the stories she was assigned: a press conference, a crime, a disaster. And then, over time, because of skill and dedication, she was permitted to pursue the stories that spoke to her heart. She didn't want to write about the president or the mayor; she decided to look instead at the lives of the disenfranchised, the needy, the elderly, the very young. *Newsday*'s circulation area is more often associated in the public mind with good fortune than hard times. But in prosperous towns, Lauren sought out the poor. Among the golden children, she found the ones who had been abused or neglected. In the Hamptons, she wrote about the homeless.

Then one day, at a hospital in upper Manhattan, a story chose her rather than the other way around. She didn't have to look far for the details; it was happening all around her, and inside her as well. Exhausted, her upper arm swollen, she went to a doctor and learned, at age thirty-six, that she had lung cancer. And eventually she decided to write about it.

"Life, with Cancer," her column was called, and it detailed what happens, first when we are sick, then when we know we are going to die. As she had from the beginning of her career, Lauren not only mined her own experiences but connected powerfully with readers. Thousands and thousands responded as she wrote with humor about the dumb things people sometimes say to those who are ill, with anger about the complicity of tobacco companies, with understanding about the challenge loving someone with cancer can pose for family and friends. She did not want to mythologize or candy-coat her experience; "Most of the time," she said, "I am scared to death." She rejected talk of heroism; she wanted readers to understand the everyday difficult life of someone who knows her life will probably be short. She wrote about the meds, the indignities, and finally she wrote about how the doctors had given her two to three months. Not long afterward, she died. The final stories carried her name but not her byline; they were obituaries that talked of the gift she'd given readers through her columns.

And that might have been the end of it.

Except that, as Lauren knew, every story is actually many stories. When she covered the TWA air crash just off the Long Island coast, she would have realized that there was the story of the cause of the crash, the story of the rescue and recovery efforts, the stories of those killed, and the stories of those left behind to mourn and remember.

This book is that last kind of story, of mourning and remembrance. Over the years, their only child taught Frank and Ginny Terrazzano that it was important to pay attention and to write things down. Lauren taught her parents by example that one way to deal with those things that cannot really be dealt with is to describe them in words. "I need you both to be strong for me," she told them after her diagnosis.

This is her father's sign of strength, his account of the life of the woman he calls "my Lauren." She didn't live long enough to write her own book; he has done it for her.

—*Anna Quindlen*

One

Dark Thoughts in a Season of Light

*W*ith the help of loyal readers from Uniondale to the United Kingdom, I have tried to hum along with my life, writing about issues from humor to the high cost of cancer. But death is a topic I've largely avoided.

It would be so much easier not to write about it. In fact, it'd be a lot easier not to think about it. Note that the name of this column is Life, with Cancer. The emphasis is on "life."

But there it is sometimes. The fear of death keeps me up at night, or it wakes me at 4 AM and I listen for a sound, any *sound outside, like a truck going by to remind myself I am still here.*

As a reporter, I've written hundreds of stories about people's deaths. I've made a career of asking uncomfortable questions with the hope of making sense of it all. Yet since that otherwise ordinary, sunny August day in 2004—the day of my diagnosis—my ability to ask the tough questions about my own life has somehow disappeared. I find it hard to ask any of my doctors how much longer they think I have.

I can't bear to know, because to put a time frame on it will somehow taint the time I have left. Still, I am frequently haunted by this question I cannot bring myself to ask out loud.

Most people are afraid of death. Yet we're all dying, a wise editor once told me. We're just doing it on different time schedules.

In my darkest moments, I worry about the future without me. First I worry about the grief of those I will leave behind. I wonder what people will say about me at my funeral. I wonder if I will be there in some way to hear it.

Grief fades with time. It's the feeling of loss that seems to linger—the little, daily reminders that a person is no longer around.

—From *Newsday*, "Life, with Cancer,"
December 26, 2006, by Lauren Terrazzano

1

The weather that late March day started out somewhat typical for this part of New England. It was chilly and blustery, but it became gradually warmer as the day wore on. The town's coastal location usually brought overcast skies and damp, saturated air, but not this day. The clouds melted away and the high ceiling seemed to produce an updraft of warm air. Perfect kite-flying conditions. By the time we arrived at the beach with the kite, it was all I could do to keep it from setting off on its own.

I strode haltingly along the sandy shoreline to allow Ginny to keep pace. My wife, a retired administrative assistant with the Tewksbury Police Department, had always been active, but in recent years she had been suffering from autosomal dominant polycystic kidney disease (ADPKD). This genetic disorder, which amounted to chronic kidney failure for which a transplant would eventually be required, caused cysts to form on the internal organs, where they frequently rupture. ADPKD also affected her liver, but my wife made the forty-five-minute car trip with me to the Cape and never complained. It was not easy for her, physically or emotionally, but she battled the pain and fatigue because she wanted to be there. We walked side by side in silence and in no particular hurry, looking for the ideal place to set the kite aloft.

Scusset Beach in Plymouth, Massachusetts, was not open for the season yet, and the shore was completely deserted. The tide was out and the coastline extended far and wide in both directions, the vastness of the Atlantic disappearing beyond the eastern horizon. We had the whole beach to ourselves.

Accompanied only by the sound of breaking waves and the occasional shriek of a seagull, I allowed myself to be distracted momentarily by the peace and tranquility of the scene in anticipation of the crushing swell of emotions that the launch of Lauren's memorial kite would evoke. It was the first birthday our daughter was not there with us.

It was hard to believe that it had been almost a year since we lost our precious Lauren to lung cancer. The grief was still there, every part of it—especially the anger. I was mad at everyone. I was mad at the world. Ginny would tell me that I needed to talk to someone about it, but I didn't think I needed anyone else telling me that I *had* to move on. Besides, I had moved on.

The day that caused me to suddenly question my faith and changed my outlook on life forever was September 4, 2004. It was Labor Day weekend. Ginny had recently begun to experience swelling and often severe pain in her abdomen and the doctors were still trying to determine exactly what was causing these symptoms. She had been seeing a surgeon, a liver and kidney specialist at Tufts Medical Center in Boston, Dr. Richard Rohrer, with whom Lauren had been in frequent contact to try to find out what was going on with her mom. Lauren had grown comfortable enough with him from their many conversations to confide in him that she had recently been diagnosed with lung cancer. Before she ever told her mother and me, she asked Dr. Rohrer if he had any suggestions as to the best way to break the news to us. She was concerned for us, not knowing how to explain it to us without worrying us to death.

He suggested KISS: Keep It Simple, Stupid.

Lauren called us during the week and said she was coming home for the weekend. We always looked forward to her visits. Lauren drove up from New York and arrived in the early evening. We were attending the fortieth wedding anniversary party for our good friends Larry and Patty Giangregorio, and we were not home yet, so Lauren let herself in with her key and waited for us. When we arrived, I gave her a hug and a kiss—and I instantly got the feeling that something was wrong. She just didn't seem like her usual jaunty self. She seemed nervous, and she looked uncomfortable. But I think what really stuck out for me was that she had not greeted me with her usual, "Hi, Oompa." It was a salutation she had begun using in jest because I had gained some weight in recent years, especially around the midsection. She always worried about my health and eating habits, so she would tell me that I looked like an Oompa Loompa from the movie *Willy Wonka and the Chocolate Factory* as a way of reminding me to take better care of myself. I always laughed when she said it because it reminded me of how much she used to love that movie. When she was young, I would sit with her and we would watch it together every time it was on TV.

But that day, instead she walked her mother and me into the living room and asked us to sit down. She sat first, dropping down hard onto the love seat, almost as if she could not hold herself up any longer. We sat directly across from her on the matching couch: it was part of the living room set Lauren had given us when we first moved into this fixer-up in Hull, Massachusetts, three years before.

Lauren looked from me to her mother several times, peering at us in deep concentration. Like me, Lauren usually got straight to the point, but this time she paused interminably. At least it felt that way. I can't help but think now that she was trying to hold in memory this image of us before we were fundamentally changed by the news she was about to deliver.

"What's wrong?" I demanded to know.

She leaned forward and reached across the small oval coffee table that was between us and touched one of each of our hands with her own. Her skin was warm and damp. "Everything is going to be okay," she began. Her words were measured and her tone was even and calm. She meant to reassure us, but it had the opposite effect. Both Ginny and I began to panic immediately.

I jumped to my feet. "Did somebody do something to you?" I flushed with anger at the thought of someone trying to harm my daughter. I knew she could take care of herself, so for her to come to us with anything could only mean it was beyond something she could handle herself.

"No, Dad. There's something I need to tell you both. Please, just have a seat."

I sat back down beside Ginny on the couch. I had no idea what the news could be, but I knew it had to be serious. We knew that Lauren had been experiencing some unusual swelling in her right arm and was planning to make an appointment with her doctor, but at this point we did not know if she had done so. To be honest, it never entered my mind that the news she was about to deliver would have anything to do with her health.

"It's going to be okay," she repeated, and I thought I detected something in her voice that made me wonder if she was trying to convince herself at the same time. She paused momentarily. Then, as if she could no longer hold it in, she blurted, "I have lung cancer."

I felt like I'd been hit with a baseball bat. Time seemed to stop. I wanted to say something, but I couldn't seem to form a coherent thought. I looked at Ginny to confirm if she had heard the same thing I just did. The frightful look on my wife's face told me that she had. Her complexion had paled and she was shaking her head almost involuntarily.

I turned to Lauren. "You don't smoke," were the first words out of my mouth, wanting to invalidate the doctor's diagnosis right then and there. I knew there had been a period several years ago when Lauren would have a cigarette on occasion, but that was it. She told her mother recently that she hadn't bought a pack since just after 9/11, and I couldn't remember the last time I'd seen her smoke. My mind was racing, and I just couldn't catch up. It just did not make sense to me that someone who rarely smoked would develop lung cancer, particularly at such a young age. I knew plenty of people who were much older, who had smoked their entire lives, and they didn't have lung cancer. I understood, as my wife did, what this diagnosis meant; I'd quit smoking myself in 1990 when my friend and neighbor developed lung cancer and died soon afterward. I knew what this disease did to people.

"Oh, Lauren!" Ginny screeched. She sidestepped the coffee table, practically leaping over it to get to Lauren, who tried to stand before her mother reached her. She was too slow, however, and they both fell back onto the chair in an embrace. I saw tears flowing freely from both their eyes and that started me sobbing.

I reached for some tissues on the coffee table, offering the box to Ginny, but she didn't want to let go of Lauren. I dabbed my eyes and walked over to them. I put a hand on Lauren's shoulder.

"What did the doctor say?" I asked after a moment, the shock still lingering. "What does he think should be done?"

"Are they sure that's what it is?" Ginny asked as she pulled back slightly, but still holding onto Lauren. "Did you get a second opinion?"

Lauren nodded. "I wanted to be sure before I told you. When I went in to have the swelling in my arm looked at, they did a CT scan that revealed a mass on the right side of my chest against my lung, and a smaller one inside the lining. I met with a chest specialist, Dr. Raja Flores, a thoracic surgeon at Memorial Sloan-Kettering Cancer Center in New York. He confirmed it."

Ginny moaned loudly as she continued to sob, pulling Lauren closer to her again.

"I need you both to be strong for me," Lauren said. "I'm going to be fine. Dr. Flores is the best there is. He thinks he can get it all with chemotherapy and radiation. And he will remove the lung if he has to."

"How soon before they begin?" I asked, gathering myself.

"They want to start the treatment right away. First chemotherapy, to try to shrink the tumors."

Up until then, Lauren had maintained her composure, but her voice had begun to tremble and her eyes welled with tears. "I was making plans for your fortieth wedding anniversary in November." Her breathing became shallow and rapid and she started sobbing heavily. Her mother held her tighter. She struggled to continue speaking. "It was supposed to be a surprise. I'm not going to be able to do it now because I'm going to be in the hospital."

I wrapped my arms around the two women I loved more than anything in the world. "Don't worry about some silly party," I consoled Lauren, who seemed more concerned about how her diagnosis would affect us than about herself. "You're all that matters. We'll be with you every step of the way; don't worry about anything."

"Yes," Ginny said. "We love you more than anything."

"I know," Lauren said with a smile. "I love you both. I feel good. We're going to get through this."

She acted remarkably brave, but I knew she was scared. I tried to be strong for her, at that moment and all through her illness.

Watching my daughter suffer through the rigors of cancer treatment over the course of the next two and half years gave me a true comprehension of just how much I loved her. Along with my wife, she was always the most precious thing in my life, but the fear of losing her gripped me tightly and would not let go. In my darkest moments, I wondered if I would succumb from the sway of this profound dread even while she was fighting for her life. It tested my strength continually.

There were times when I would look at Lauren while she was asleep or resting after a treatment, or other times when she was feeling better and talking with her mom, and suddenly my mind would become besieged with memories, reminding me of things I thought I had forgotten long ago.

The reality was that I could not even be sure they were my

memories. I worked a lot when Lauren was young, putting in long hours, so I would rely on Ginny to tell me how they spent the day and she would fill me in on all the details.

2

Katy Greer was four years older than Lauren, but from the time Lauren was a baby, the two girls were as close as sisters. To Katy, Lauren had always been Laurie. Nobody else ever called her that, but that's how Katy would address her into adulthood.

The Greers lived on the same street we did in Everett, a small, mostly middle-class city just north of Boston. Katy had an older brother and an older sister, and Ginny and I got along well with their parents. In 1972, the Greers moved to the town of Tewksbury, situated about fifteen miles north-northwest of Everett. To the two girls it may as well have been a thousand miles, because they never thought they would see each other again. Then one day we went to visit the Greers, and I was immediately taken with the quiet, pastoral setting. The community was much smaller and more rural than I would have thought. I also noticed that the house right next to the Greers was available, so I inquired about it.

Land was something that I had always held in high regard. Land was at a premium close to Boston and just too expensive. But just a little farther away from the city, you could purchase a home and a considerable plot of land, often multiple acres, for a reasonable price. Like many proud Italian Americans, I fancied myself if not a farmer, then at least a glorified gardener. My parents and grandparents always had a little vegetable garden, even in the city. If there was room enough for a couple of tomato plants, maybe some zucchini or eggplant, every inch of that little plot of earth would have something growing in it. And even if I couldn't make something grow from the ground, just having enough dirt to move around was something that was very appealing to me.

Our entire lot size in Everett was 3,200 square feet, so when I saw that the house next to the Greers in Tewksbury was on a full acre (a whopping 43,560 square feet), I had to have it. Fortunately, convincing Ginny to move was not as difficult as I imagined it would be. Lauren had not started school yet, and we would not be all that far from Boston. Best of all for Lauren, she would have Katy right next door, even if there was an acre of land between our houses. Suddenly, I was a farmer.

Lauren was four years old and Katy was eight when we moved to Tewksbury, and despite the age difference, they were always together, playing and growing up in a sprawling, safe neighborhood with woods all around and lots of other children. Katy would often come to our house to play with little Laurie. She would carry Lauren around like a big doll, which we thought was very cute. Lauren was always tiny. Katy, who was the baby in her own family, pretended Lauren was the younger sister she never had.

Katy was over a lot. The girls would play with Barbie dolls for hours on end or run around with our dog, Benji. Watching television was the other mainstay. I remember how much Lauren loved *The Flintstones*. We had an organ at our house, and Lauren would try to teach Katy how to play *Spanish Eyes*, a song I played for her. After playing together all day, Katy would often have dinner at our house. I would be late quite often for those meals, or miss them entirely.

On the weekends, however, when Katy was over, we would all do things together. In the summer I would take the girls for ice cream, and on Sundays Katy would sometimes come with us when we would visit my mother and father in East Boston. Lauren's grandmother and grandfather liked Katy a lot. One of the dishes my mother always made for the girls was eggs and potatoes; she cooked them together rather than having eggs with home fries on the side. It was not something Katy got anywhere else, and she loved it.

Something else all kids like to do is swim. Katy had a built-in pool, and Katy's mom taught Lauren how to swim. The girls would attend each other's birthday parties and put on little shows, mostly just being silly and laughing. I recall one Easter when Lauren slept over at Katy's house and the Greers left an Easter basket for Lauren to find when she woke up in the morning. They'd spread powder around the basket and made tiny bunny footprints in it to create the illusion that the Easter Bunny had visited the house during the night. Lauren was so excited by that. She talked about it for weeks afterward.

As a child, Lauren was quite shy. In second grade, before making her First Holy Communion (a rite of passage in the Catholic Church), she was supposed to make her first confession, which was the sacrament of reconciliation, and receive her penance, but she was terrified and did not want to go to confession. Ginny was having a tough time getting her dressed and ready, but Katy was there, and she somehow found a way to ease Lauren's mind and talk her into going. Ginny was very grateful.

My wife got along very well with Katy, who had become as much like a daughter to Ginny as a sister to Lauren. Katy used to like to brush Ginny's hair, which she perhaps did so often because Lauren did not like anyone to touch her hair—especially her mother, who was always trying to braid it or put it into a ponytail or pigtails when she was a little girl. Lauren would resist, preferring to let it grow wild and perhaps more than anything delighting in defying her mother. It was something that I admit to taking some secret pleasure in myself. I taught her to speak her mind and be straightforward at all times, so I took pride in my daughter's displays of her convictions, even if it was at the expense of my wife, though it was just as often at my own.

As she got a little older, Lauren was afraid to walk home alone, especially if it was getting dark, so Katy would accompany her to the end of the driveway and watch as Lauren ran like the wind down the street and up her own driveway, yelling to Katy all the way until she was safely inside her own house.

By the time Katy started high school, their age difference began to affect the girls' relationship. Their interests started to vary, and they naturally drifted apart. Katy was getting her driver's permit while Lauren was still playing dodgeball with the younger kids in the neighborhood. For a while, Katy would come around for special events, like when Lauren went to her proms, and take pictures of her younger friend. But as time went on they went their separate ways, Katy building a life for herself and her family in Massachusetts and Lauren establishing her journalism career in New York. Not surprisingly, the girls saw less and less of each other, and then lost touch completely for a short time.

Katy was surprised when she first learned that Lauren went to Boston University, a big-city school; that choice didn't seem to reconcile with her memory of the shy little girl who could not make it to her house next door without a chaperone. The girls later reconnected in 1988 when Katy got married. Lauren was a maid in her wedding. When Katy traveled to New York with her husband and parents to be our guests when Lauren walked down the aisle for the second time, Katy was impressed by just how much Lauren had changed over the years. The shy young girl Katy had played with was now a successful journalist in a traditionally male-dominated profession. Katy, a small-town New England girl and new mother, was amazed to see that Lauren had everything under control and organized; she took care of everyone, even making sure that Katy and her family got into a cab and the driver knew precisely where to take them. Katy told me later how impressed she was that Lauren had come so far in so many ways. Laurie had become Lauren.

3

Every time I looked at Lauren, those kinds of memories would flood back. Maybe it was because I did not want to see just how sick she really was, wanting instead to remember her in happy times. Lauren put on a brave face for us, but I knew my daughter, and I knew her well enough that she could not mask what she was really going through. Looking back now, I often reflect on a particular moment that Lauren and I shared, when she revealed to me just how frightened she was; she looked to me to make it all better, and I could not. The memory haunts me still.

During those terrible days when Lauren was going through her cancer treatment at Memorial Sloan-Kettering Cancer Center, Ginny and I would stay with her in New York. She had a small co-op apartment on the Upper West Side of Manhattan, just a block from Central Park. The chemotherapy made her terribly weak and ill, and we would stay to comfort her and help her do the little things she had trouble doing for herself. We would clean, prepare her meals, make sure she was getting the proper nutrition and plenty of rest, and basically just spend time with her. We spent the weekends and as many weekdays in New York as we could. The treatment often made her nauseous, and she frequently was not able to keep food down. I sometimes held her head while she vomited, keeping her hair out of the toilet. Her mother and I did our best to make her comfortable, much as we did during her childhood when she was sick. But this was so different. I wasn't prepared. Far from it.

One night, Lauren was quite ill and vomiting frequently. She was unable to sleep and I asked her to sit with me. As I held her in my arms on the living room couch, she looked up at me, wide-eyed and helpless, and asked, "Daddy, am I going to be all right?"

She looked so small and vulnerable; she might have been ten years old again.

"Yes, sweetheart," I said. "Everything's going to be okay. I promise. Just try and get some rest."

She smiled and put her head on my shoulder. My reassurance made her feel better, even though she knew better. We both did. Those were just words. But I wanted to believe them myself more than anything. I wanted to believe that just saying so would make the cancer go away.

It was a difficult reality for me to come to terms with. My daughter was confronting the uncertainty and terror of a cancer diagnosis. As a father, I wanted to protect her and do everything possible to make things all right. It was instinctive. How could I tell her the truth, and at the same time accept that there was nothing I could do? Cancer was something that only her doctors and modern medicine could defeat. Her ultimate safety was out of my hands, and I felt completely powerless at a time when she needed me most. It was a debilitating feeling for me, but I did not want to cause her any further worries, so I tried my best not to let her see my feelings of helplessness. I would cry later, at moments when Lauren was not around to see me, the tears falling freely from my eyes. There were times I didn't think they would ever stop.

I learned a lot about Lauren during that difficult time. The way she handled the diagnosis and the subsequent treatment made me realize just how courageous she really was and how committed she was to her responsibility as a journalist. But I really didn't know just how strong she was until April 2006. After a brief period of remission, her doctors found the cancer had returned near her ribs, and they immediately performed surgery to remove the tumors. Soon after, she decided that she was going to document much of her personal life and her medical progress in a weekly column in *Newsday* titled "Life, with Cancer." She convinced her bosses of the idea that others could learn from her experiences, and she was right. The response from readers was overwhelmingly positive. I was never more proud of her. She investigated the disease the same way she did any other story she was writing, and she shared her knowledge with the rest of the world. Before then, I thought I knew something about lung cancer, but it turned out I knew very little. In a short period of time, however, I learned quite a bit about it. And I learned it all from Lauren. It was a bitter education for her also, as she became a teacher as well as a student.

4

I carried the kite with Lauren's picture on it farther along the beach and then suddenly stopped. It was time to let it go. Something told me this was the spot, and I prepared to launch the kite.

I looked at the photo of Lauren on the kite, and fresh tears came to my eyes. It was my favorite picture of her. She looked so beautiful. It had been taken by one of her girlfriends at a park in New Jersey about eight months before she died. She was standing in front of a tree, her arms folded across her chest. Her eyes look as large as saucers and she has an inquisitive expression on her face that anyone who knew Lauren would have recognized right away. The 8-x-10 image of Lauren was printed onto a white sheet of paper.

The traditional diamond-shaped kite featured the photograph of Lauren across its white cover, and below it were these words: *LAUREN—IN LIFE "REACHED FOR THE STARS."* Written near the top of the left and right trailing edges were the words *"LAUREN LOVE + MISS YOU VERY MUCH!"*

As I readied the kite for its inaugural launch, so many memories came back to me. It wasn't just her illness and her death that preoccupied me. Her life was filled with countless moments of joy and triumph. She'd meant everything to her mother and me, but she'd meant a lot to many people, to her friends and the people she wrote about in her articles. I guess I never really thought about that to a great extent until after she died, but I see now that she had touched many lives and made them better, more fulfilling, more meaningful.

But sadness was not what this day and event was about.

Twice each year, in tribute to the life and memory of our beloved daughter, we take the special kite out and fly it in her memory: every March 28, on Lauren's birthday, then again on May 15, the day she passed. I've always felt closest to Lauren during these commemorative kite runs. I could feel her presence then and there, more than I did anywhere else.

Ginny has not always been well enough to make the trip with me, but that first time, she was by my side. She was weeping as she reached out and touched Lauren's picture.

"Lauren," I said, "our force of love, light, and life. We love you and miss you very much." Then I set out running slowly back down the length of beach we had just traversed. The kite rapidly ascended, the wind taking up the line faster than I could feed it out, almost pulling the reel from my grasp. There was a break in the cloud cover above, and peeking through was a swatch of azure sky, a color reminiscent of Lauren's own beautiful blue eyes. It seemed to beckon the kite ever upward. I truly felt her spirit with us.

When Lauren was a little girl, we would fly kites together for hours on end. I would sometimes take her to the park or a local schoolyard, but mostly we went to a quiet little beach on the north shore in Revere, not far from our home in Everett.

She loved it, as did I. Kite-flying had long been a hobby of mine, and I had built quite a collection of kites through the years. There was something about flight in general that I always found fascinating. Sharing my enthusiasm with my young daughter was fun for both of us.

I could still see her little feet running barefoot through the sand as she followed the flight of the kite gliding across the sky, her tiny faced flushed with excitement as she screamed, "Daddy, Daddy, make it go higher! Make it go higher." She could not contain her exhilaration as she reached her arms up toward the ascending kite, a trait that would remain part of her very being—always reaching for the sky in all her endeavors in the thirty-nine years that she was with us.

Lauren was always precocious and determined, and her mother has to be given much if not all of the credit for how Lauren turned out. She devoted herself entirely to our daughter while I was away providing for my family. I put in fourteen-hour days for many of those years. I worked my way up from purchasing, production planning, and scheduling at Louise's Home Style Ravioli Company, one of the largest manufacturers of Italian pasta products in New England. I would come home late, very tired, and I often had to eat dinner alone. So Ginny was home with Lauren during the formative years, making sure she did her schoolwork and instilling in Lauren a love for literature and writing that would become the basis for her later career in journalism.

However, besides giving her an early introduction to kiting, I like to claim that I inspired Lauren with my own enthusiasm for photography. She was fascinated by it, and she was a natural. Lauren had a genuine eye for visual composition. She became quite an accomplished photographer, which complimented her skills as a journalist. I think she surprised herself when some of her photographs were chosen for exhibition in a genuine New York City art gallery.

5

Lauren carefully boxed up the last of the framed photographs and then let out a sigh of relief. All the pieces were ready for the short excursion over to the Long Island gallery the next morning. Eden Laikin, Lauren's good friend and colleague at *Newsday*, was by her side. They had been chatting and sipping merlot, but to celebrate Lauren's first photo exhibition, Eden popped the cork on a bottle of champagne and poured two glasses. They both giggled as sparkling wine fizzed up the flute and spilled down the sides.

"To Lauren's new career as a photographer."

"I don't know about that," Lauren said, "but I've gotten pretty good at framing."

"To Lauren, the picture-framer!"

The girls laughed as they clinked glasses and took a sip of champagne.

Eden told me she could see that Lauren was excited but also nervous. Lauren's journalistic endeavors had always won her praise and awards, but more importantly she saw the real results of her writing, with many of her stories facilitating changes to some of the more outmoded and abusive practices within the social welfare system.

Her photography, however, was something she was not quite as certain about. She was proud of her photographs, but she did not know how they would be received.

"You did a remarkable job," Eden said. "You could have picked any twenty. They're all that good."

Lauren was dismissive of the praise, but Eden thought the pieces were truly extraordinary. There was a story behind each one. The color, sepia, and black-and-white photos, including some multiple-exposures prints, perfectly captured the essence of the women and children from a Guatemalan town that had been devastated by deadly mudslides the previous fall.

"What drew me to these beautiful Mayan women," Lauren said of her attraction to the subjects, "was that they seemed to have very difficult lives, yet they seemed so strong. I think I was looking for symbols of strength."

She had taken hundreds of photographs, twenty of which were being featured in a photo essay on display at Fotofoto Gallery in Huntington, on the north shore of Long Island; that was where the framed photographs needed to be delivered early the next morning. Eden offered the use of her large SUV to transport the pieces, and she stayed over that night to help Lauren get them ready.

Lauren had recently moved into the one-bedroom co-op apartment on the West Side. It was actually quite roomy compared to her previous one in the same area of Manhattan. The apartment was bright and cheerful and Lauren loved everything about it. The ten-story building had a doorman in the lobby and was a block away from Central Park, where Lauren jogged prior to her cancer diagnosis.

Eden knew that Lauren did not like having anyone living above her, so she was not surprised to see that Lauren had chosen the uppermost floor. When Lauren was a freshmen at Boston University, she lived on an all-female dormitory floor, while on the all-male floor directly above were several Palestinian students who were quite heavy on their feet. They were also musicians, and whenever they practiced, the sound reverberated through the ceiling and shook the walls. On occasions when Lauren was trying to study in her room and they were stomping around above her head or rehearsing their music, she would end up going upstairs and politely asking them to quiet down. Eden had heard Lauren tell that story on numerous occasions, but Lauren always downplayed one significant aspect of her action. She was undoubtedly polite in imparting her request, so it might not seem like such a big deal, but when you consider that she was reprimanding young men who came from a very different culture, one that was misogynistic in many ways, her request must have shocked them. At the very least, they would not have been used to being talked to in such a way by a woman. But they did not know Lauren, and she certainly got their attention. What started out as a contentious situation became a mutual friendship over time as the loud students living above Lauren came to respect her, not in spite of the way she stood up for herself but because of it.

Lauren always got along with everyone. Her dorm at BU was like a miniature United Nations. She had roommates and friends from all around the world. In fact, Lauren's photographs and the gallery in Long Island that exhibited them had been an indirect consequence of one of the international friendships that she made later on while attending graduate school in New York.

A year earlier, Lauren's cancer was in remission and she was feeling good, so she made plans to travel to Guatemala to visit Dina Fernandez, a classmate and friend from Columbia University who was now living in her native country and working there as a journalist. When Hurricane Stan struck Central America a week after Lauren arrived, Guatemala was hit the hardest of all the countries in Stan's path. Lauren managed to travel to several remote regions that had been devastated by deadly mudslides and offer her assistance, employing both her journalistic and photographic skills in documenting the disaster. This was a big, breaking news story, and Lauren seemed to be in the right place at the right time.

Now, not quite finished celebrating after the bottle of champagne was empty, Lauren treated Eden to dinner at a little Italian bistro that she enjoyed not far from her apartment. It was a nice night, so they walked to the restaurant and sat at a table outside, where they continued the conversation they had started earlier. They were quite close, and no subject was off-limits, but it was one of the first times that Eden remembers talking to Lauren about God and her faith.

Though Lauren had been brought up Catholic, receiving all the sacraments and attending Mass on Sunday, she wasn't a particularly religious adult. Eden told me that her friend seemed to feel that God had forsaken her, maybe even that she was being punished for something. Eden told Lauren that her God was not a punishing one.

"God doesn't make bad things happen," Eden said. "Bad things happen and God helps us through them."

Lauren remained unconvinced of this, and Eden further explained that her own faith was the one thing that got her through even the largest of struggles in her life.

Lauren knew that Eden had lost two very close friends in the past couple years, and that Eden had been with them right up until the final hours of their lives. Eden never hid her esoteric belief in mediums that could communicate with the dead. She felt she had been chosen, in some way, as the person who was supposed to be with those friends so that they could have someone to talk with about dying and about their fears and doubts. As hard as it may be for most people to have such conversations, Eden came to discover that it was something they all really wanted. And needed. And now Lauren was asking.

Eden admitted that she, too, had personally struggled at times with her faith. She told Lauren that she could not understand why such a thing was happening to someone like her.

"But you know," Eden said, "it doesn't matter what the doctors say or what any of the tests show, because they're not God. Even if they think they are. If you're supposed to live, you will."

She told Lauren that God doesn't give us more than we can handle. Lauren scoffed at the cliché, but thanked her friend for all her support. It had been a long day and they were both tired. They went back to Lauren's apartment and crashed.

The next morning they got up bright and early, loaded the photographs into their vehicles, and headed for the gallery. On the way, with Eden following in her SUV, Lauren got a flat and had to pull over to the side of the road to change the tire.

Lauren cursed to herself as she rolled down her window. "God doesn't give you more than you can handle, huh?" she yelled to Eden. "Now I have cancer *and* a flat tire!"

"Maybe," Eden responded, "we're not supposed to be on the road yet, not for another twenty minutes. Maybe there's going to be a major, horrible accident on the FDR and God wants to delay us in order to save us."

Lauren's response was to roll her window back up without response, but Eden could see her laughing through the windshield.

6

Lauren had always been adventurous, spirited, and tenacious. The very traits that helped make her an outstanding journalist sometimes drove her mother and me crazy. When she was a young girl we called her LT, which she naturally thought was because those were her initials, but in truth it was shorthand for "Little Terror." Even as a child, Lauren wasn't afraid to show how strong and clear she felt about what she wanted.

Leah Ritchie and Lauren had grown up about a mile from each another and went together through grade school and eventually high school in Tewksbury, Massachusetts. The girls first met in kindergarten, but it was actually in third grade that they became the very best of friends. Back then, Lauren used to think that Leah looked like Kermit the Frog, but one day at recess in the little playground at Shawsheen Elementary School, Lauren approached Leah, looked her up and down, and said, "I think we should be friends." And that's what they were from that day on.

And like the friend Lauren picked for life that afternoon, it seemed her career ambition was also something that had been determined early on. Lauren made it clear enough to Leah that she wanted to be a journalist. Around the same time, Lauren started her own little personal newspaper, writing some stories that were apparently of interest to third-graders and distributing them to her classmates. Whenever she had a new edition to get out, she would run down to the basement and pull out a beat-up old automatic typewriter we kept in a basement closet. There was always an imagined deadline, and I could count on having to put some time into the repair of a stuck key, frozen carriage return, or broken ribbon. You could see Lauren's determination even when she was a little girl, her tiny frame leaning over the typewriter, taking her time and precisely striking each letter with all her strength.

Leah can still explicitly recall how, during a field trip to Lexington Battle Green, the memorial park in Lexington that was the site of the opening shot of the American Revolution in 1775, the teachers were looking for Lauren after all the other children were aboard the bus and accounted for just before they were ready to head back to school. Lauren was found not far away with camera in hand. It was an expensive camera, one of mine that she liked to use to take pictures of animals and scenery. That day she had wandered off to get a picture of something that interested her. Being in the moment, in the experience, and capturing what was going on, was the most important thing—more important than her own personal safety. Lauren was fearless that way.

Leah told me about another time when she was being bullied by a girl at school, a girl who was much bigger and taller than she was. When Lauren found out what was going on, she announced to Leah,

"I'm going to have a talk with her." Lauren, who was of even smaller stature than Leah, did go and talk with this bully, and although Leah never knew what Lauren had said, the girl never bothered Leah again.

I was not surprised when Leah told me this story. Lauren was not a hero, nor was she especially brave, at least by any standard definition. She was fearless, however. And that was something she demonstrated from the time she was a very young girl. The summer when Lauren was ten, we vacationed in Lake George, a resort area in the Adirondacks in northern New York. The first day I rented a speedboat, and before we even got it in the water, Lauren asked me if she could drive it. I hesitated, but she continued to insist. I thought if I took her out on it and she saw how fast it really went, she would back down. That didn't work. In fact, she wanted to pilot the craft more than ever. With just a minimal amount of instruction, she operated the boat better than I did. I was with her, of course, to make sure she was safe, but she exhibited no fear. Same thing when I took her skiing for the first time. I used to be an avid downhill skier, and I introduced Lauren to the sport at a very early age. Before long she was going down the intermediate and expert trails with me. She was absolutely fearless. It didn't matter if it was roller coasters or bullies, she was not afraid of anything.

Two

To the Rescue

I knew I was in love the first time I saw him. He barely had any hair and walked with a slight limp. When I looked into his brown eyes, he acted as if he wanted to crawl under a table. I always seem to go for the complicated ones.

The workers at the New York City animal shelter said he was found scrawny and scared, wandering the Hunts Point section of the Bronx.

I wasn't looking for a dog. I am 38, newly married, and sufficiently scarred from a seemingly endless tango with a disease that has led me through chemotherapy, surgery, radiation, a brief remission, more surgery, two more rounds of radiation, and more chemotherapy. All in 25 months.

But while people credit me with rescuing him, a few sage observers know it was really the other way around.

In fact, so intrigued are cancer researchers by the role of pets in patients' lives, the National Institutes of Health is studying whether dogs have any impact on alleviating pain and anxiety during treatment. It has long been known that having a pet is therapeutic on a number of levels, for everyone from autistic children to the elderly. And even if adoption isn't an option, most shelters have volunteer programs that allow people to be part of an animal's life.

Still, the dog came with his own baggage. His teeth were bad, his ears were infected, he was matted with tar and oil, and he had a bad cough. Someone theorized that he had been living under cars or big trucks.

Nobody could guess what breed he was, this particular dog.

—From *Newsday*, "Life, with Cancer,"
March 6, 2007, "What Cancer Gives: Anger,
Not Wisdom" by Lauren Terrazzano

1

Some little girls love their pets. Other little girls collect stuffed animals. Our little girl collected pets—animals of all kinds, actually. Officially, she only had one dog, a miniature schnauzer named Benji who was part of the family for seventeen years. Lauren treated it like a sibling, dressing it up in doll clothes or her own clothes. And whenever she found animals that were injured or lost or needing help of any kind, she would pick them up and take them home. She would have kept them all in her room if we had let her. Some were in need of rescue, and she would take them in to try to nurse them back to health. Then, when she thought they were healthy enough to make it on their own, she would set them free or we would bring them to the local animal shelter. For a while, I thought for sure Lauren would end up being a veterinarian when she grew up.

Early on I realized that it was just in her nature to help. Lauren had a great appreciation for life at an early age. She seemed to reach out instinctively whenever she witnessed suffering, and she'd try to do something about it. One time when Lauren was no older than seven, she took action to save a wild rabbit that had fallen into the clutches of a neighborhood cat. She chased the cat away and scooped up the suffering animal. There was no blood or any other sign of physical injury, but the bunny appeared hurt and was certainly scared. Lauren brought it into the house, where she and her mom nursed it back to health. The animal survived the ordeal, and it was this experience, I believe, that helped Lauren realize how much of a difference she could make by taking deliberate action, by getting involved in something outside of herself. In those tender years, she was only in a position to help pets and other animals in peril, but as she grew and later began her career as a journalist, she clearly possessed the same regard for human life and dignity. This was apparent as her concern turned toward the welfare of those less fortunate who lacked a voice in society. For Lauren, it was never political or religious but more a moral responsibility and social consciousness. If she felt it was the right thing to do, she acted on it.

I don't recall having ever made an actual connection between that little girl who chased away the cat to save the rabbit and the woman who advocated for the human rights and dignities of people by writing about children who were abuse victims, elderly people who had been exploited and neglected, and other people who could not defend themselves. At least this was not a correlation I made until after Lauren's death. That was when it suddenly became very obvious to me, but because I was a card-carrying liberal, Lauren's work as a journalist had always been a source of great pride for me.

2

Lauren was a great friend. She established lasting relationships with people, and her girlfriends were an integral part of who she was. The bonds that she formed with them were so strong that her friends became kind of an extension of her. They remained close to her throughout her life and I know that meant a lot to Lauren. They were all there beside her right until the end, and that meant so much to her mother and me.

Three years before they began working together at *Newsday*, Jessica Kowal met Lauren when they were graduate students at Columbia University's journalism school (J school). Jessica learned a lot in the program, but one of the most valuable lessons came from Lauren's example. While still a student herself, Lauren coached Jessica and other future journalists on just how a reporter should go about finding a story, even if he or she was looking in another direction entirely.

As part of the two-semester program at Columbia, Reading and

Writing 1 was a fundamental course in which the students were introduced to the craft of journalism. It was in this class that Jessica and Lauren first became acquainted. Every Monday the instructor, Robin Reisig, gave the students a different writing assignment that covered one of the basic types of stories that journalists might be expected to report on in their careers. One week they were asked to write a "court" story, which required them to go to a courthouse and develop a story from what they observed. The assignment seemed straightforward enough. Lauren went to night court in Manhattan, which basically was arraignment court. It was usually very busy, with a new case coming up every few minutes in which a judge decided if a defendant was to receive bail or not.

At this criminal-justice assembly line, Lauren noticed that there were children, some very young, who had come in with their families. The parents were there because their teenagers had been arrested and were being arraigned, and younger siblings had been dragged along.

Some of these children were sleeping on the hard wooden benches or curled up on the cold marble floor beneath. Others hadn't eaten any dinner, feasting instead on concession stand cookies and orange-flavored soda.

"On a busy night," one court officer told Lauren, "we see twenty to thirty kids here." He described how some would run unsupervised around the lobbies, taking bad falls on the marble floors and hurting themselves.

Certainly everyone saw the children there, but no one really noticed them. Lauren did, and this became her story. While the other graduate students focused on what was happening with an individual case in the courtroom and were busy interviewing the judges and lawyers, Lauren talked with the families: the parents, who were going through a very difficult time, and the children, who had themselves become inadvertent victims of the court system.

Lauren focused part of her story on a six-year-old boy who had been clutching a Barney lunchbox as he tried to sleep on his grandmother's lap alongside his two-year-old brother. The boy's grandmother told Lauren that the older child was terrified by the whole ordeal and just wanted his mother (who was in court to post bond) to come home. It was already 10:00 AM, and the family would end up waiting a total of fourteen hours before the mother was arraigned on a simple assault charge after a fight with a former boyfriend.

The boys' grandmother told Lauren they could not afford a babysitter and expressed her frustration and concern for the welfare of her grandchildren. "They're going to get sick," she told Lauren. "It's freezing in here and look at what they are exposed to." She pointed toward the front of the courtroom, where two tuberculosis and hepatitis-infected defendants in surgical masks were waiting to be arraigned.

"We see people in here with tuberculosis, meningitis, and hepatitis," another court officer told Lauren. "I wouldn't bring my kids here."

Lauren learned that the courts had some slight provisions in place for taking care of children in this situation, but those provisions were clearly not adequate. She reported that the New York City Family Court was the only provider of daytime care to kids who were either witnesses in cases or defendants' children, and that the parents in criminal and civil courts could go to the Family Court center for child care only during the day, when it was usually overcrowded.

There was, however, a state judicial commission that had begun looking into establishing a number of pilot centers around the city that would act as referral centers for social services agencies to determine if the children were eligible for programs such as Medicaid and Head Start.

"We want to get them outside of the courtroom and into a care program in that difficult time," the commission's cochair told Lauren.

More than just the children's discomfort was at issue; the welfare of not only these children but all other children in the future who would inevitably find themselves in that courtroom or one just like it somewhere else really bothered Lauren. She became personally involved in the story, and by writing about it, she identified a real problem and asked the court system and the public to get involved, to do something about it. The story she ultimately wrote revealed how those families lived and struggled together with the associated problems of being in the criminal justice system, and it all came as a result of Lauren noticing young children in the courtroom struggling to stay awake while waiting for a family member to be arraigned.

The approach that Lauren took on this story helped Jessica understand the difference between reporting, where you file a story using facts and information gathered from interview notes, and real journalism, where you actually look deeper into a subject to find a story that may not be as obvious.

Jessica was amazed that a student her own age could possess such an insightful journalistic eye. Jessica wasn't the only one impressed. The story was accepted for publication by *Newsday*, the paper where

Lauren would one day work, and it ran as a "Closeup" feature in the New York edition on November 8, 1993. It was the first story Lauren had published in a major newspaper, and she was still in journalism school.

As they worked together in subsequent years, Jessica observed that Lauren's strength as a journalist never deviated. She observed firsthand Lauren's innate quality to consider humanity first as she explored the human experience by revealing what people face in their daily lives and showed that changes could be made to make life better for the people in her stories. She shared with me that Lauren seemed to possess a core belief that was based on a profound respect for each human being and how life should be lived with dignity. Jessica observed this in the newsroom watching Lauren work on a story, and it was something that came through time and again in the stories Lauren wrote. She would actually feel offended and hurt personally if people were mistreated, so her mission as a journalist became the desire to help change and improve people's lives.

Jessica learned a lot from Lauren about journalism and also learned a lot about Lauren from her journalism. Lauren didn't just report a story; she lived it. Jessica felt it took a certain fearlessness to delve into something unpleasant with the goal of coming away with something positive where a lesson could be learned and an improvement could be made. That was what Lauren did.

3

Robin Reisig came to know Lauren in three different contexts. Robin was one of Lauren's professors when Lauren was a student at the Columbia University Graduate School of Journalism. Years later, they taught a class together at Columbia when Robin asked Lauren to take an adjunct teaching job at her alma mater. The two women also became friends during that time. Lauren spoke often of Robin and always spoke very highly of her. Robin taught her a lot, and as I would find out years later, there were also lessons that Lauren had for Robin.

As a student, Lauren very much stood out among her peers. Robin regarded Lauren, Dina Fernandez, and Jessica Kowal to be the three strongest reporters in the class, but Lauren was a rare student. Robin often described her as indefatigable, a terrier who would grab onto a story and not let it go. She had seen students work hard and develop into first-rate journalists, but Lauren was a born reporter who was infinitely curious and saw so much beyond the obvious. She followed up on everything she did, and then followed up on that. Robin expected great things from Lauren early on.

Over the years, Robin had seen Lauren's "court" story become elevated to an almost mythical status around campus, with instructors who never knew Lauren repeating the story to motivate students to dig deeper and go further with a story and Columbia journalism school grads talking to each other about it as if it had happened in another era. But there was more to the story that few people outside of Lauren's closest friends and colleagues ever heard about.

After *Newsday* accepted Lauren's story, the editors requested that an accompanying photo run with the article, and Lauren was asked to go along with the photographer. They visited a young mother and her small child in their apartment. While inside, Lauren saw something stamped on the walls by the New York State Department of Health. The notice warned: "Health Hazard—LEAD PAINT—Must Be Removed Immediately." The stamp was several years old; Lauren learned through her background research of the story that at the time the warning was first posted, a small child living in the apartment had recently fallen ill and had been diagnosed with lead poisoning. The owners of the building never removed the hazardous material or did anything else to make the place safe. The landlord didn't even bother to hide the stamps on the walls; the apartment was just rented to another family with small children. Lauren ultimately discovered that this residence was a public housing apartment building run by the New York City Housing Authority. Her observation resulted in a second story about children in public housing and the lead paint problem, a story which she started working on immediately.

Robin also taught Lauren the following semester. In the Newspaper Workshop, the students who were interested in editing the *Bronx Beat,* the school paper, took turns at the helm. Robin asked Lauren to step in and edit the paper for a while because of some ongoing issues with the staff. Initially, Lauren balked at the request. She just wanted to focus on her reporting; that was the only thing she ever wanted to do. Becoming an editor was the last thing on her mind. However, when Robin explained that she was in a pinch and needed her, Lauren reluctantly agreed, and ended up doing a remarkable job filling in.

One of the first things Lauren did when she was in charge of the *Bronx Beat* was to expand the paper to twelve pages. While that might not seem to be such a big deal, it had always been eight pages, and the change not only took guts but required imagination. Lauren had to come up with enough quality story ideas to make it work and be successful. During her tenure as editor, Lauren also established the newspaper's first photo page. She thought the school-run publication looked too much like a newsletter with only eight pages and no photographs. She felt that the improvements would increase circulation as well as give the contributing student-journalists more exposure and more confidence as a result. She knew how hard her classmates worked on the stories and what it took getting them to print. They were important stories and they needed to be read.

Robin praised Lauren for her editorial decisions, though Lauren ended up doing even more of the work on the paper as a result of her displeasure with the effort put forth by the student who had been tasked with editing the photo page. Lauren would do that job as well, and it came out brilliantly. The entire edition, actually, was so good that Lauren won the prize for the school's best editor that year. But even after having great success editing *Bronx Beat* and winning that award, she had absolutely no interest in ever working as an editor. In fact, the day she walked up to receive her prize, Robin noticed that Lauren made almost no attempt to hide the scowl on her face. Robin had to laugh when Lauren's name was called, because seeing Lauren grumpy was not something anyone often saw.

After receiving her postgraduate degree at Columbia, Lauren stayed in touch with Robin. She would call periodically just to catch up or to ask her former instructor for professional advice about reporting. Sometimes she'd ask Robin's opinion on something she was working on, which she often needed reassurance about in one form or another. Robin saw this as another example that revealed how dedicated Lauren was to her craft, always demanding more from herself, even if she was frequently overly critical of her work. Robin followed Lauren's career and was aware of how much Lauren had been able to accomplish so quickly. Yet at the same time, inexplicably to Robin, Lauren continued to harbor a lot of self-doubt. It is said that great reporters and writers have a brooding insecurity that causes them to continually check and double-check everything to be sure nothing is overlooked. In that sense, it is their insecurity that fuels their greatness. That was certainly a quality that Robin recognized in Lauren, as did her mother and I. Lauren always expressed doubt. Even in grade school and into high school, after she took an exam that she was well-prepared for, she was convinced that she had not done well. Yet when the test scores came in, her marks would be among the highest in the class.

Being an adjunct instructor at the Columbia University Graduate School of Journalism is more demanding than at many other journalism schools. It is also somewhat unusual; the core curriculum at Columbia is taught by two professors. One has to be a full-time faculty member and the other is required to be a working journalist. While both professors are allowed to choose an adjunct, the selection must be approved. When Robin asked Lauren to assist her for a summer term, she agreed immediately. I remember that she was very excited and honored to be a part-time faculty member at Columbia.

Robin remembers that Lauren brought a lot of energy and enthusiasm to the classroom, and the students seemed to really respond to her. She was so good and she enjoyed the interaction with the students so much that Robin recommended her to other faculty members.

As a teacher, Lauren was always well prepared. In fact, in Robin's opinion, Lauren was overly prepared. For example, for one class Robin asked her just to participate in the class discussion about finding story ideas as an investigative reporter, and Lauren proceeded to give a forty-five minute lecture on the topic. Robin realized that this simply reflected how much Lauren expected of herself.

After teaching together, Robin and Lauren gradually became dear friends. Unfortunately, that burgeoning relationship was short-lived because of Lauren's subsequent diagnosis with lung cancer. But Robin was never more proud of a student than she was when Lauren began her "Life, with Cancer" series. Like thousands of other people, Robin read Lauren's column each week in *Newsday* and was deeply moved by her writing. The candor and humor Lauren used to relate the human experience of living with a terminal disease touched Robin as a person, as a woman. The honesty and courage Lauren showed in putting a public face on a highly stigmatized disease certainly opened up many eyes, including Robin's. She told me that she'd always thought highly of Lauren, but the columns made Robin fully appreciate what a force my daughter was, a light that shone so brilliantly even in a sky full of stars.

And just like that, the light was extinguished. Robin felt the void when Lauren lost her three-year battle with lung cancer. In the

remaining years that she continues to teach, Robin says she is waiting for the next Lauren Terrazzano to come shining through . . . but
she knows there will never be another.

4

M onica Quintanilla was working as a reporter at the *New York
Daily News* in the Queens bureau when she met Lauren in
1994. Monica had been working as a journalist for about ten years
but had only been at the newspaper a couple months when Lauren
arrived to begin a one-year internship at the paper. Monica knew
from the moment of that first encounter that they were destined to
become dear friends.

Early one morning before many people were in the office, Monica
walked into the newsroom and saw a bright-eyed, energetic young
woman who gave her a broad smile. Lauren introduced herself, and
the two women started a dialogue that would last until Lauren ultimately lost her battle with lung cancer.

From the beginning of their acquaintance, it was apparent to
Monica that Lauren was a very determined journalist who worked
extremely hard and wanted to have a real impact with her work. She
learned what I already knew: it was important to Lauren that she
establish her reputation in the field.

Monica and Lauren had many things in common besides work.
They shared a similar zeal for life and adventure. One of the things
they liked to do whenever they had the opportunity was go out
to dinner. Lauren wasn't a big eater, but she enjoyed going out to

restaurants with her friends, and she didn't care if the group was big or small. She didn't care if the restaurant was trendy or the most expensive; she wanted to have the best that particular restaurant had to offer.

In New York, you can eat out every night and never dine at the same restaurant twice, no matter how long you live in the city. Lauren learned quickly where the best places to eat could be found. Whatever type of food or particular dish someone expressed a desire for, she could come up with a list of choices for any budget. I liked to say she was a walking, talking Zagat guide.

Lauren and Monica liked to laugh and have fun, and the two friends were constantly on the phone with each another when they weren't together. Several calls a day were normal, but they would chat even more often on occasion. Later, they would sometimes drive to work together. Monica lived in New Jersey and would pick Lauren up on her way in to Queens.

Lauren did very well as an intern that summer, but she was not asked to return to the paper for another year; that wasn't unusual, even for interns who perform well. Not being offered a position had nothing to do with her performance or ability, but Lauren was very upset that she had been overlooked. She was also experiencing the added pressure of her pending marriage.

Monica advised Lauren to apply to other area papers, so she circulated her resume to just about every newspaper, big and small, in greater New York and New Jersey. She soon received a job offer from the *Bergen Record,* a northern New Jersey daily that was the second largest paper by circulation in the state (after Newark's *Star-Ledger*).

Lauren was initially excited by the opportunity that presented itself so quickly; the paper was fairly large and situated not far from Manhattan, which made her commute from the Upper West Side quite convenient. However, Lauren was not there long before she began expressing her discontent, stating in no uncertain terms to me and anyone else who would listen that she did not like it there. In fact, she would tell Monica that she hated it. It was unusual for Lauren not to get along with people, but she did not seem to click with her coworkers. She found that the personal and professional culture at the *Record* was quite a bit different from the one she had gotten used to in her brief time at the *Daily News*. There was a fierce and distrusting competitiveness among the staff at the *Record* that made Lauren uneasy. By comparison, the veteran reporters and the newbies, as well as the interns, all got along exceedingly well at the *Daily News,* and that was where she really wanted to be.

Lauren was so upset that she considered taking time off and leaving the *Record* so that she could study Spanish in Guatemala. She went so far as to investigate several Spanish immersion programs there because she believed that being able to speak Spanish would be of great benefit to her as a reporter as well as give her a distinct employment advantage over other journalists who might be in competition with her for a job at a major newspaper.

This attitude led indirectly to a conflict between Lauren and Monica. It was actually part of an ongoing problem involving what Monica perceived as Lauren's disinclination to send her resume to *Newsday.*

This was around the time that *Newsday* was closing down its New

York edition. While *Newsday* has always been very much a Long Island–based newspaper, for years it also had a completely autonomous New York edition with its own editors that operated as if it was a separate newspaper. That edition had once been very competitive with the other city papers. Staff was located in the main offices in the city as well as in satellite offices that operated out of smaller branches in the other boroughs. In fact, there was as much competition between *Newsday's* Long Island and New York editions as there was between *Newsday* and the other major papers. Because the New York edition became too expensive to operate, it was closed in 1995. Only the office in Queens was left operational, staffed by a skeleton crew. Queens was the largest of the five boroughs in land area and that branch was the only one that the newspaper's publishers felt had any chance of selling copies.

Because of *Newsday's* cutbacks, there were a lot of journalists out of work at that time, and Lauren believed there would be no way she would get a position in that field of competition. She figured she needed to cut her teeth by writing for a smaller paper for a while. She also believed that the *New York Times* and the *Wall Street Journal* were not real options until she'd learned her trade and begun to make a reputation for herself with her work.

Monica disagreed. She argued for Lauren to apply to *Newsday* for the very same reasons that made Lauren hesitate. Monica believed that many of the displaced reporters working out of the defunct New York offices would not want to go work in Long Island, and they wouldn't want to work for their old nemesis. In her opinion, many of the most talented journalists were likely to seek jobs elsewhere, both

in state and out of state; some would land on their feet with prestigious magazines, and some would simply retire altogether. For this
reason, Monica thought Lauren had as good a chance as anybody in
nailing down any position that became available at Newsday.

But Lauren just continued to complain about the Record and how
much she did not like it there, refusing to put in for a position at
Newsday. Monica knew that Lauren had been doing very well at the
Record and had written some compelling stories in her short time
there. It was time to make a move. However, nothing she said could
convince Lauren.

Lauren's incessant whining about how much she disliked being
at the Record finally got to Monica. She completely changed gears.
Instead of mentoring Lauren on the topic and being sympathetic
and supportive, Monica sternly chastised her friend, telling her to
stop complaining and just make the best of it. She added that Lauren
need not bother to call her again until Lauren's resume was sent to
Newsday. This little edict was clearly figurative in nature, and Lauren
knew that it was not meant to be taken in the literal sense. But it
seemed to work, because not long after that confrontation, Lauren
phoned Monica and excitedly informed her that she had received a
call from Newsday after sending in her resume; they'd asked her to
come in for an interview.

Over the next few days, Lauren learned everything she could
about the newspaper that was considering her for a job, including
its history, readership, and key personnel. When she went to the
offices in Long Island the following week, she impressed the editors
with her enthusiasm as well as the ability she had shown while at the

Record. They asked her back for a tryout, and when they offered her a job, she accepted it, amazed by the starting salary it included. At the time, *Newsday* was the seventh largest daily in the country.

Lauren was extremely happy and excited. She knew she did not have to say anything to Monica for her help in making it all happen, but she did anyway. She thanked her friend for her tough love and support, and then she treated Monica to dinner as a token of her gratitude.

It was early 1996, and Lauren was covering the town of Brookhaven to begin her career at *Newsday*. However, Lauren being Lauren, that was not enough. Besides her beat, she took every other assignment she could get, and from the start she was logging a slew of hours. She was even traveling and freelancing.

Her first real travel assignment for the paper was to Pennsylvania to cover the bizarre story of John E. du Pont. The millionaire and chemical fortune heir had been arrested by police after a two-day standoff and charged in the shooting death of Olympic wrestler David Schultz. The murder took place on du Pont's eight-hundred-acre estate, which he had turned into a camp for professional wrestlers. Lauren was a young reporter on a high-profile case; she did a great job with it, a fact that did not go unnoticed by editors or colleagues.

Right from the start, Lauren loved everything about working at *Newsday,* including all the people she worked with. She was very happy and finally felt complete as a person. This was not something Lauren ever stated overtly, but it was plainly observable to Ginny and me just how content she was with her professional career and her life. It was satisfying for me as well because as any parent knows, when your child is safe and happy, there's no better feeling in the world.

A year later, Monica left the *Daily News* and joined Lauren on the staff at *Newsday*. This was about the time Lauren decided that what she really wanted to do was cover social issues. She was so dedicated to her job she could be found in the newsroom most days by 7:00 AM and would often stay there until midnight. It was a hectic pace that would have run anyone ragged.

I knew Lauren was a hard worker who dedicated herself fully to everything she did with the same intensity. It was something I encouraged and respected. Of course, she had a tendency to edit the things she told me and her mother so we wouldn't worry as much. Fortunately, we had Monica. Acting as a parental stand-in, she cautioned Lauren, advising her to take some time off to relax and be with her husband Peter. He and Lauren had gone on a number of hiking and camping expeditions together, and it always seemed to do Lauren a world of good, allowing her to clear her head and forget about the newsroom and deadlines for a couple days.

5

Lauren met Peter Gabriele on an Amtrak train bound for Providence, not far from where he grew up in Smithfield, Rhode Island. He was coming in from New York to visit his family and Lauren was continuing on to Boston to see us. They started a conversation and found that they had a lot in common. He was three years older than Lauren, but they came from similar backgrounds and were close to their families. They ended up talking for a long time. Peter was interested in seeing her again, and she felt the same way.

At that time (spring 1992), Lauren was writing for the fashion industry trade journal *Women's Wear Daily,* sometimes referred to as the bible of fashion. From talking with Lauren briefly, it became clear to Peter that this was not what Lauren wanted to be doing. She would not only do the stories that were required of her, but was always looking for something more than what her editors were expecting, perhaps presenting a topic from a completely different perspective or putting a unique spin on a story.

They exchanged numbers and went out on a few dates when they got back to New York. By the end of 1992, Lauren and Peter were still seeing each other. Professionally, Lauren had moved on, taking a position with *Traders Magazine,* an industry publication that provided news and information on anything having to do with financial trading. She became an associate editor, writing cover and feature stories on trading-room technology and reporting on Securities and Exchange Commission rulings and their impact on the NASDAQ market. She also wrote and edited the monthly "Industry Watch" section. This subject matter happened to be right up Peter's alley as a Wall Street stockbroker.

However, this was not where Lauren wanted to be either. And she wasn't there long. While completing her master's in journalism at Columbia University, she wrote for the *Bronx Beat,* a student-produced weekly newspaper, covering educational and general-assignment stories. Peter observed that during this time, Lauren seemed to take her signature journalistic ability of digging deeper and going further with a story than anyone else to a new level. Peter knew couples in New York who would go out for a drive just to get out of the city for a while, but it was not that easy with Lauren. She was always looking for a story. When Lauren was behind the wheel, it became even harder for the couple to escape for a change of scenery.

One afternoon she drove them to the Bronx and began cruising through the neighborhoods to look for something to write about. She didn't have an assignment due; she was just looking for a story. Another time, Lauren had read about an industrial waste controversy involving a business facility operating in a Bronx neighborhood. Peter ended up riding around with her for the better part of the day as she questioned some of the people living in the area about why they would allow this kind of plant to operate in their backyards where their children played. Nobody seemed to think it mattered, but it did to Lauren.

Her compassion was one of the many qualities Peter loved about Lauren, and when he asked her to marry him, she seemed as overjoyed as he was that they were engaged.

Ginny and I both loved Peter from the start. He was a great guy, ,and we thought he was wonderful for Lauren. As he and Lauren spent more and more time together, we got to know him well. He and I would go out for lunch together whenever he came up to visit Lauren. We both liked to eat, especially enjoying hearty Italian meals. There was a particular restaurant in nearby Everett where we would go for tripe, something we both really loved.

Lauren and Peter were married in the summer of 1995. I gave my daughter a big wedding with all the frills. Two hundred fifty guests filled the reception hall at the Lennox Hotel in Boston to witness Lauren and Peter exchange their vows. She had so many friends there, and it was a nonstop—borderline raucous—party that lasted all night. Everyone seemed to enjoy themselves that night, especially Lauren, and that made me feel good. That's what it was all about.

Starting a family was something they had discussed, and it was something that they both wanted very much. I admit, Ginny and I were both overjoyed by the prospect of becoming grandparents. However, these newlyweds were every bit as married to their careers as they were to each other. They were both ambitious, and they were young relative to their professions and how much time it takes to attain a certain level of achievement. I knew that Lauren's work was never far from her mind. She put in a lot of hours, and I could see how that might put off a new husband. In this case, it was a detriment that went both ways: Peter was a nine-to-five employee at J.P. Morgan and went out frequently at night with clients and colleagues.

When the two of them were able to get out of the city for a little while together (while they were dating as well as after they were married), they usually spent the time in the wilderness on hiking and camping adventures, from locations from upstate New York to halfway across the world. They would throw on their backpacks, toting little more than some basic provisions, a tent, and sleeping bags, and leave the world they knew behind for a couple days at a time. They went on many memorable trips together, but for Peter the excursions that most stand out were the ones in Idaho and the Canadian Rockies on the American side of the spectacular mountain range.

On their honeymoon in Hawaii they hiked the Kalalau Trail; from vistas stretching up more than 4,000 feet from the Pacific Ocean, the trail provided a spectacular view of the Islands. To stand amid lush greenery while all around incredible waterfalls cascaded down from the etched mountaintops to the valley floor was an experience beyond comparison.

Their trip to Guatemala in 1995 was something quite special as well. With Lauren, no trip meant visiting just one or two places; she had to see everything. She had to visit all the little towns and hard-to-reach villages. She wasn't happy until she took in every experience that she could. Lauren was that way about everything, not just travel.

A real turning point in their relationship came on July 17, 1996, the day of the TWA Flight 800 crash off Long Island. Peter believed that the catastrophe had a profound (and detrimental) impact on Lauren and marked the beginning of the end of their marriage. It was during Lauren's reporting of the disaster for *Newsday* that they started to noticeably drift apart. It wasn't just the fact that the stories occupied her so completely for so long, consuming many weekends and cutting into the only time she and Peter had to spend together. The experience seemed to change her in a fundamental way. Peter noted that she had become more serious, more intense, focusing even more strongly on her work. But what was perhaps most harmful to their future was Lauren's sudden shift in thinking about starting a family—she no longer seemed to have any interest in having children. Becoming a father, however, was still something Peter very much wanted, and this conflict divided them deeply.

Peter saw how the crash of Flight 800 affected Lauren. She cried more easily. She would talk to him about the tragic loss of life and question why something like that had to happen. She learned so much about many of the individuals—particularly the children who perished—that it was as if she had known them personally. She had seen their personal effects floating in the water—a stroller, a toddler's toy, a child's backpack. She would tell Peter and some of her friends that she sometimes had a difficult time getting those images out of her head.

Although it had been a difficult assignment for Lauren, she visited and talked with members of many of the victims' families and ended up writing some of the best features of her career. That was no coincidence; she identified with those people, closely sharing their pain and anguish. Long after the crash investigation was completed, Lauren stayed in touch with the families, sending cards during the holidays and calling on the anniversaries.

One of the stories that had a major impact on Lauren involved a woman whose fiancé perished in the plane crash. He was carrying an engagement ring with him and he intended to give it to this woman later that summer. Recovery divers found the ring floating in the water amid the debris. It was still in its silk box from the jewelry store where the couple had purchased the 1.6-carat diamond together. It took almost until Christmas that year, but the FBI finally returned the ring to the woman for whom it was intended.

Peter believed that Lauren suffered a significant degree of trauma as a result of her immersion in stories such as these, and together with everything else she saw and experienced during the course of the reporting she did on TWA Flight 800, her trauma impacted both their lives. Whether her behavior could have been attributed to a condition such as post-traumatic stress disorder (PTSD) Peter does not know, but whatever the case, the plane crash seemed to alter Lauren's perspective on life. She was never the same again.

On several occasions I talked with Peter, as well as Lauren, about the problems they were having. To me, it seemed their fractured relationship was reparable, and I urged them to go to counseling together. Peter was willing to try it, but Lauren did not even want to consider it.

I really noticed how far apart they had grown during a trip the four of us took to Italy and France in October 1998. Lauren had planned the entire trip more than a year in advance, and it included stops in Provence, Nice, and Cannes on the French Riviera, and Monaco. It was all so exceptionally beautiful, and I was amazed at my daughter's proficiency in the French language. But Lauren and Peter hardly talked, and it was obvious that something was wrong. Lauren spent a lot of the time shopping and doing things with her mother, and she was cold and distant with Peter when we were all together. It was sad to see them split, but because she was so unhappy, her mother and I gave her our full support, and we all had to say good-bye to Peter. By early 1999, their marriage was over.

6

One of the "Life, with Cancer" columns that generated the most feedback was the one Lauren wrote about the dog she adopted from a local animal shelter. It was actually the very first installment in the series. One of the reasons Lauren decided to begin the series that way was because she knew people always seem to respond to positive animal stories. I remember the day Lauren adopted the dog; she called us with excitement and told us all about him and how he had come into her life.

She had just left Memorial Sloan-Kettering Cancer Center in Manhattan that afternoon after receiving radiation treatment. She was feeling well enough to walk and ended up on East 110th street, between 1st and 2nd Avenues, where the Animal Care and Control Center (AC&C) was located. AC&C is the largest pet organization in the northeast; they rescue, care for, and find homes for nearly 40,000 homeless and abandoned animals each year.

Lauren described how she walked into the shelter without any forethought. All the dogs began barking at once. There were so many it was deafening. She told us how she noticed the one dog that was not making any noise and was cowering in his cage with his head down, which instantly caught her attention. She said she knew right then that she had to have him.

"I found Bartufalo," she said to the shelter worker with a smile. That person did not know what Lauren was talking about, but we did: during her recent travels through an isolated region in northern Italy, she spotted an old man picking walnuts in an open field and stopped to chat with him. Bartufalo was the name of the friendly old dog by his side. Lauren loved the name so much she adopted it for the one dog at the shelter that she just had to have.

The most accurate description of the American version of Bartufalo (Bart, for short) might have been "mangy little white dog." The exact breed or combinations thereof was anybody's guess. When

Lauren first saw him, Bart was in pretty bad shape. Attendants at the shelter had found him wandering the Hunts Point section of the Bronx, an area known to be pretty rough. His fur was spotty from being shaved to remove clumps and tangles. (Lauren joked that she identified with the animal because she had no hair either.) What little tufts of fur remained were filthy and splotched with tar and oil. He had a terrible cough and a limp. His teeth were bad and his ears were infected. He had probably survived by sleeping underneath cars and trucks and rooting around garbage cans eating discarded bits of food.

But when his fur grew back, he was actually cute. He ate everything in sight, even if it wasn't something digestible. He was a street dog, but he was lovable. Lauren did everything with the animal, including bringing him with her almost every time she came to visit us. She seemed to most enjoy taking him with her on her daily walks in Central Park, which she did right up until she became too weak and could no longer go herself.

Three

Cancer Rises Amid Smoke and Mirrors

I smoked off and on for about five years, not really the profile of the typical smoker who developed the disease as a result of her bad habit.

Still, the new marketing push seems doubly sinister, especially upon learning that the hugely profitable tobacco company hosts "girls night out" events with makeovers and free packs of cigarettes to get women interested in the brand.

A long way from one of those parties, I sat last week in Room 1428 of Memorial Sloan-Kettering's lung cancer ward, where I am being treated at this point for the symptoms of the disease after a nearly three-year fight. I was trying to get in touch with Camel's marketing guru, the man who came up with the strategies to lure women to smoke Camel No. 9.

In an interview last week, the company's marketing expert, Craig Fishel, characterized the campaign to reach women, plainly and simply, as "an opportunity." But he insisted, "We're not targeting young women," because he said the tobacco company won't advertise in a publication that has less than 85 percent adult readership, which is defined by the demographics as age 18 and older. "It encapsulates all adults," he insisted. I insisted that 18 and older means young women, the same ones who were drawn to the Glamour magazine that featured the Camel No. 9 ad and a cover shot of Drew Barrymore this month.

Thirty percent of its Camel brand smokers are female. The new cigarette made its debut in February, right as Congress began to debate sharply limiting tobacco marketing.

To be fair, I do have mixed feelings on this issue. I believe in free will when it comes to smoking. We have all made decisions about it at one point or another.

But I wonder if a teenager or a 20-something woman reading the magazines has the will power to stay away from cigarettes, as she is simultaneously bombarded in

*neighboring pages with messages about being thin and
how to lose fat.*

*The fact is, Joe Camel should take a hike. A very
long one. In the desert.*

—From *Newsday*, "Life, with Cancer,"
April 17, 2007, "Cancer Rises Amid
Smoke and Mirrors," by Lauren Terrazzano

1

I was angry. Extremely angry. When it completely settled in my brain and there was no question remaining that Lauren had cancer, I was filled with inexorable rage. I didn't know how to deal with it. I desperately wanted to do something, but I was frustrated by the fact that there was really nothing I could do to rid my daughter's body of that disease. I never tried to hide my anger (not that I could), but Lauren had remarkable success with calming me down when put to the task. She seemed to possess an innate ability to temper my mood in the same way she was able to soothe other people in times of stress. On one occasion, she managed to pacify me from across the expanse of the Atlantic Ocean.

Lauren and her mom, Ginny's father and sister, her sister's husband, and her uncle Al were on their way to Italy. They had been talking about taking this trip for a long time before it finally worked out, thanks to Lauren. The morning of departure was Friday, May 27, 1988. Everyone was very excited. Both of my parents had health concerns, and I didn't feel comfortable leaving them for an extended period of time, so I stayed behind.

It was a bright, sunny morning as they left for the airport. Ginny could not wait to get there, in part because flying made her nervous. Sleep was out of the question, so she spent the time talking with Lauren and occasionally looking out the window at the Atlantic Ocean. The rest of the family was seated in another section of the plane. As they made their way over the Bay of Biscay, with Spain visible outside the right cabin windows, the plane suddenly began to descend. Not sharply, but it was obvious to Ginny that something was not right. By this time, Lauren was asleep next to her. It was about 7:00 AM French time, and they were not scheduled to land for two more hours. They were approaching the French coastline and Ginny began to see the topography of the region, the vineyards and châteaus of the great Bordeaux region.

Just then she saw a flight attendant trying to get the attention of another attendant. He signaled the woman with a thumbs-down gesture and Ginny's stomach sank along with the flight pattern of the plane. The sleeping passengers awoke to the sound of the pilot's voice over the intercom announcing that they were in the process of making an emergency landing. The passengers were asked to adjust their seats and fasten their safety belts. No reason was given for the situation, but whatever it was, no one on board felt it could be good.

Moments earlier, unbeknownst to any of the passengers, Alitalia officials in Milan had received a threat from a caller claiming that a bomb had been placed aboard the jumbo jet. Within minutes, Italian police contacted authorities in France and the FAA instructed the plane to land immediately.

On board the aircraft, no one spoke. Lauren reached out and clasped her mother's hand. The flight attendant explained that they would be landing shortly at the closest airport, about 220 miles southwest of Paris. There, they were told, they would have to exit the plane by sliding down the emergency chutes.

Ginny looked over at her sister and her father.

"It's going to be all right," Lauren said.

The flight attendants immediately went to work, the word "bomb" escaping from their lips as they scurried about the cabin. Ginny was in shock, disbelieving what she was hearing.

"Don't worry," Lauren reassured her mother. "Everything is going to be fine. Just listen to the flight crew."

Once the Boeing 747 aircraft was on the ground, the passengers and crew had to be evacuated as quickly as possible. The chutes that the 398 passengers were instructed to slide down were thirty to forty feet off the ground. Ginny and Lauren watched the rest of their family exit the plane ahead of them. Ginny saw her eighty-six-year-old father disappear down the chute, cool as a cucumber, with his arms raised straight up into the air. When it was Ginny's turn, she paused and looked down and saw how far down it was to the tarmac and felt a tug of panic. She told me later that couldn't get herself to slide down.

"Mom, we have to get off," Lauren told her. "You can do it."

Ginny felt a slight nudge at her back. It was my Lauren, and before Ginny was fully ready, Lauren gave her a little push and down she went. She closed her eyes and slid to the bottom, and Lauren followed close behind.

The passengers were told to run as quickly as they could, to get as far away from the plane as possible. Once they were at a "safe" distance, Lauren gathered the family together to check on everyone. Everyone seemed okay except for Ginny's uncle Al. He had injured his leg during the evacuation, and though it was not serious (a moderate ankle sprain and some swelling around his knee), he did not continue on to Italy but returned home to the United States.

As they proceeded to the terminal building with the other passengers, they saw that a number of other passengers had been injured as well. This was a time long before cell phones, and Lauren searched for a public phone to try to call me; she knew that if I heard about the bomb scare on the news later that morning, I'd be a basket case. But she was told that she would have wait until she got through customs. By the time she got through to me, it was about three in the morning. I answered the phone half asleep.

"Dad, don't worry," was the first thing Lauren said. "We're all fine. Everyone is okay. Mom's fine. She's right here beside me."

She explained what had happened, and I felt an instant rush of relief just from talking to her. I had every confidence that Lauren would take care of her mom and the family. As she handed the phone over to Ginny, her instincts as a journalist kicked in. She spotted an Italian journalist she'd met on the plane and asked him if she could borrow his camera. She had checked her camera with her bags and did not have access to it.

Lauren proceeded to photograph the entire scene, including the plane on the tarmac with the forty-foot chutes unfurled and the evacuated passengers inside the terminal looking tired and confused.

She tended to her family, making sure they were comfortable and had everything they needed, but she also spoke to other passengers. Lauren was fluent in both French and Italian, so she became the interpreter not only for her family but some of the other passengers as well. She documented the entire ordeal, which lasted more than ten hours, as security searched the plane and all the luggage for explosives. The bomb scare turned out to be just that—a scare. There was no bomb, but for Lauren and Ginny and her family, and probably every other passenger aboard the diverted Alitalia flight to Milan, the stress of travel coupled with the stress of the bomb scare had taken its toll. It was nearly another two hours of flight time before they touched down in Milan, but no one could relax.

Needless to say, I could not get back to sleep. The next morning I spent hours trying to gather as much information as I could from the local and national news broadcasts and called all the Boston media outlets—newspapers, television, and radio.

I got another call early that evening from Lauren, who reported that they had all made it safely to their final destination. She was excited to be in Italy. She said it was the most beautiful place she had ever seen and that the weather was perfect. She told me she would have it all documented for me in a series of photos albums that I could look at when they returned.

I got the opportunity to visit Italy the following year. Lauren was majoring in communications at Boston University, with a concentration in art history and Italian. Before embarking on her career, she wanted to experience the Italian culture more intimately than the pages of her textbooks could offer. After the December semester in

1988 she transferred to Trinity College in Connecticut in order to take part in an exchange program in Italy. She studied in Rome the following semester, and Ginny and I arranged a trip to meet her in Rome at the end of the spring semester in 1989. We flew into Zurich and went on to Italy from there, joining a train tour traveling through the Alps and the Swiss countryside before stopping in Milan, Venice, Florence, the Tuscany region, and then finally Rome, just as Lauren's semester ended. We spent four days with Lauren in Rome, then we all went together by train to Salzburg, Austria, the home of the von Trapp family; Lauren was infatuated with *The Sound of Music*. We stayed there overnight before heading back to Zurich for a couple more days, then returned home together. It was the most remarkable trip—the beauty of the countryside and the cities was unlike anything Ginny and I had ever seen before. Being in those places and experiencing them with Lauren at that time was the best part of all.

2

On July 17, 1996, Lauren had been with *Newsday* about four months when one of the worst aviation disasters on American soil occurred just off the coast of Long Island.

Just after 8:30 PM, twelve minutes after taking off from Kennedy Airport, TWA Flight 800 suddenly exploded and fell in pieces into the Atlantic Ocean. The wide-bodied Boeing 747 was bound for Paris with 230 passengers and crew aboard when it blew up 13,800 feet above the ocean, just ten miles south of Moriches Inlet.

The night of the crash, Lauren was dining at a Queens restaurant with a number of other *Newsday* journalists and editors. It was a celebration of sorts, the staff having come out of a year in which the paper had gone through some difficult times. In 1995, *Newsday* closed its New York edition and a lot of people lost their jobs, retired, or found work elsewhere. A year later, things were starting to look up; the paper had survived and seemed to be turning the corner. Management had recently hired a group of young and talented journalists, including Lauren. Their impromptu team-building dinner was beginning to wind down when some early model cell phones started to go off. News of a missing plane and possible crash off Long Island put the journalists on high alert. Sitting among them was assistant managing editor Miriam Pawel, who immediately took charge of the situation, assigning the journalists different tasks to ensure complete coverage of the breaking news story. The journalists scattered in different directions; Lauren was sent to the beachfront. Her job was to get as close as possible to the crash site. It was about a forty-five-minute drive from Queens to Suffolk County, Long Island, and Lauren raced to the scene.

There was a lot of confusion and speculation from the very moment of the crash. Because the explosion had occurred without warning and with no emergency call from the cockpit, a terrorist's bomb or even a land-to-air missile attack was suspected to have brought down the large jet. Of the hundreds of eyewitness accounts, a couple dozen reported a flash rising from the ground just before the plane disintegrated into a fireball.

The crew aboard a New York state Air National Guard aircraft on maneuvers off of Moriches Inlet spotted the explosion and were the first responders. The National Transportation Safety Board (NTSB) was notified within minutes and a team was quickly assembled in Washington, DC, before making a trip out to the crash site the following morning. Because the NTSB does not investigate criminal activity, the initial possibility—that a terrorist bomb or missile had been involved—prompted the FBI to initiate a criminal investigation alongside the NTSB's accident investigation.

The whole area became a crime scene. The Coast Guard swiftly mobilized to set up strict security zones to keep all unauthorized aircraft and vessels out of the search area. Suffolk officials sent deputy sheriffs, town and village police, and military personnel in four-wheel-drive vehicles to patrol the beaches to discourage curious sightseers and to look for the bodies of the victims from the doomed flight. Suffolk also sent flood maps to the command center so workers could determine where the tides might be most likely to wash bodies ashore. It quickly became apparent that there was little hope of finding any survivors and that this would be a recovery mission, not a rescue.

Lauren not only made it to East Moriches but she managed to talk her way through the various blockades and police checkpoints, not to mention the backyard of a property owner who came out of his house with a shotgun, before eventually winding up inside the Coast Guard rescue center. For a period of about twenty-four hours she was one of only two *Newsday* reporters allowed in the facility.

The Coast Guard deployed about fifty cutters and other vessels, along with half a dozen helicopters, whose pilots used night-vision goggles to detect and gather plane wreckage and victims. The massive search effort was aided by numerous state and local agencies, including the Suffolk County Police Department, which put six of their own rescue boats in the waters off East Moriches, and the New York City Police Department, which sent a helicopter to the scene.

Eventually, 95 percent of the airplane would be recovered from three primary wreckage areas. These pieces were transported to a hangar at the former Grumman aircraft facility in Calverton, New York, for storage and closer inspection and, later, reconstruction. This facility became the command center and headquarters for the investigation.

The human toll was enormous. Recovered bodies were placed on Coast Guard cutters whose decks were stained with blood, then brought by smaller boats to the makeshift morgue in a Coast Guard boat warehouse, then later moved to Hangar B at the Air National Guard base in Westhampton before a thorough investigation could be made at the Suffolk County medical examiner's office in Hauppauge. Some remains were badly burned and disfigured beyond recognition. Postmortems revealed that some of the victims had drowned, though they were believed to be unconscious when they hit the water. Each body bag was opened only long enough for a photograph to be taken and to note any identifying characteristics or jewelry before they were moved to refrigerated trucks.

As family members of TWA Flight 800 passengers arrived at Kennedy Airport for information, the airline put them up at a nearby hotel overnight. There was initially no official statement from TWA; up to that time, the airline had only made public the number total of the passengers aboard the flight, a number which they revised twice before settling on the figure of 230, including 212 passengers, four-teen flight attendants, and four cockpit crew members. The airline said it wanted to notify all the families before releasing the individ-ual names.

By daybreak the area was crawling with politicians and officials from every level of state and federal government. Besides Mayor Giuliani, Governor George Pataki soon arrived on the scene, as did U.S. Transportation Secretary Frederico Pena and FAA Adminis-trator David Hinson. The Federal Bureau of Alcohol, Tobacco, and Firearms sent special agents who had expertise in explosives. From conversations I had with Lauren during this time, I knew it was not easy for her to hear all the grisly details that were being reported in the early hours following the crash. It was much later on that I learned just how difficult it had been for her. Once again, not want-ing to worry her mother and me, Lauren hadn't shared much; it was her friends who revealed to me that Lauren sometimes had difficulty getting some of the images out of her mind. She admitted to having lucid nightmares from which she woke up trembling uncontrollably. During waking hours, she thought about the victims and their fami-lies, talking about their emotional stories to the point of tears.

Lauren's biggest asset to the paper had always been her ability to get people to talk to her about an unfolding tragedy. That was the task she was given when TWA Flight 800 went down. Her job was to talk to family members who had lost loved ones on the doomed flight.

The disaster posed colossal challenges for the paper and its staff on all assignment fronts, so Lauren was far from alone. Ben Weller, a *Newsday* editor, sent a reporter to the home of one of the victims. The reporter was promptly turned away by the family. With no one else in the newsroom, Weller approached a summer intern, who grew visibly pale and noticeably nervous at the thought of having to interview a victim's family. Weller then got hold of Lauren, who was still out in the field, and gave her the assignment. Lauren went to the same household and within an hour she called the newspaper from the family's living room where she was talking with the victim's husband while looking over intimate family photographs. Forty-five minutes later, Lauren was back at the office writing about the interview she had with him.

Lauren's natural ability to win the confidence and even affection of people in difficult circumstances was a strength. Lauren realized this and used it to her full advantage. She once told me that she first became aware that she possessed such a skill while she was in journalism school. One of her professors taught her that all journalists possess unique personal strengths that can be exploited for the betterment of their craft. This was hers. She radiated a natural empathy that made people trust her, a trust she never betrayed.

3

The TWA disaster generated many different stories by different *Newsday* journalists over a long period of time. After several weeks, stories involving the victims and their families slowly played themselves out. After that, the focus became the ongoing investigation into the cause of the crash, which required an updated story every day. For Lauren, looking into what the NTSB was doing was the second phase of the work she did on the crash of Flight 800. This was when Lauren and Sylvia Adcock began working closely together, becoming two of the lead reporters on the story.

Sylvia had been handling more of the investigative aspects of the crash all along, so for the first few weeks their paths never crossed. In fact, Sylvia and Lauren did not know each other well before the crash. Lauren had only been at *Newsday* for four months while Sylvia had more than ten years experience as a journalist. In Sylvia's eyes, the few times Lauren had crossed her path, albeit briefly, she had found Lauren's peppy, gung-ho attitude a bit bothersome—pestering in a younger sister kind of way. But that all changed when Lauren and Sylvia started working together, and over the course of the next ten years the two women become the closest of friends.

At the time of the crash, Sylvia had been the transportation reporter for *Newsday*. Anything involving the streets, highways, bridges, the subway, JFK, or LaGuardia was her domain. She also wrote a regular transportation column, so when Flight 800 went down, Sylvia was assigned to the NTSB, which she really did not know all that much about. However, she would quickly learn all that she needed to know alongside Lauren during this investigation and in subsequent airline disasters. *Newsday*'s FBI journalist was also deeply involved for a while because of the initial reports that there might have been a bomb aboard. Investigators held their briefings at the Sheraton, not far from the investigation site, so Sylvia, Lauren, and other journalists all congregated there to conduct their interviews and get updated information.

The two of them also had to make several trips to Washington together as the investigation shifted focus. They were seen so often together that one of their editors began to refer to them as "Agent Small and Agent Y'all." Sylvia's southern accent wasn't strong, but it was obvious enough, and Lauren was petite, despite having what Sylvia liked to tauntingly refer to as disproportionately large feet.

Eventually, the crash investigation reached its conclusion. It was revealed that no act of terror (or a missile) had been responsible for bringing down the jumbo jet.

Out of this tragedy emerged the nonprofit support group Aircraft Casualty Emotional Support Services (ACESS), which helps family members of aircraft crash victims. Founded by Heidi Snow, fiancee of Michel Breistroff, a French hockey player who died aboard TWA Flight 800, ACCESS also conducts sensitivity and support training for airlines and other companies that regularly deal with bereaving families and crash survivors. (The American Red Cross had provided similar services for two weeks, but after that, Flight 800 families were on their own.)

About a year after the TWA 800 accident, Snow attended a support group for relatives and friends of the victims of Pan Am 103. After the meeting, she kept in touch with some of the members of the group and eventually asked them if they would mind talking to people she knew who had lost loved ones on Flight 800. She paired mothers with other mothers, orphans with orphans, fiancees with fiancees.

I recall Lauren telling me about Heidi Snow's efforts, which she fully supported. Lauren remained in contact with family members of some of the victims of the Flight 800 accident, and she advised them to participate in the support group if at all possible. It turned out to be a rousing success, and that's how ACCESS was born. Snow and her organization have since arranged meetings between loved ones of victims of many other major aviation disasters as well as those who perished during the terrorist attacks of 9/11.

4

The *Newsday* staff was awarded the Pulitzer Prize for its spot reporting of the TWA Flight 800 disaster. Lauren did not go to the Pulitzer lunch, Sylvia recalled, but she ended up attending the Los Angeles Times-Mirror Company award ceremony with Miriam Powel and several other *Newsday* journalists who could not make it to the Pulitzer lunch. Lauren was proud of what she had done, for herself and the paper, but she was not satisfied with it, meaning she was not through. She wanted to accomplish much more. Early on she often told her mother and me that her goal was to win a Pulitzer. Sylvia, too, believes that this taste of early success really helped Lauren blossom as a journalist and made her hunger for more. She could get people to open up to her as a reporter as few journalists could. She proved that to herself and everyone else with her coverage of the aftermath of Flight 800. To the people she interviewed, she was genuine and sensitive; to her editors she was competitive and aggressive. Lauren wanted to get the story before the *Times* and the *Daily News,* and she had developed a keen sense for cultivating sources and establishing their trust. As Lauren began doing aviation stories with Sylvia as well as her social services pieces, the two of them grew closer still. Sylvia observed Lauren's confidence and her work ethic one holiday season when she saw Lauren sitting at her desk in the early morning writing Christmas cards. It was still quite early in December, and Sylvia made a comment to Lauren about getting a jump on getting her Christmas cards out to her family early before she forgot or things got too busy.

"Oh, no," Lauren said. "The cards are for my sources."

Sylvia was amazed, thinking how she barely got cards out to her friends, and here Lauren was writing out detailed messages on the cards to her sources.

"One of my professors in journalism school suggested it," Lauren added. "So I do it every year."

It seemed to pay off. Not only would her sources talk to her, but they would sometimes let her know what other reporters at other papers were working on, which to a journalist was valuable information.

Over the course of the next five years, Sylvia and Lauren would work together on several aviation disasters for *Newsday,* including the crash of Swiss Air Flight 111 on September 2, 1998. The jet had departed JFK for Geneva, Switzerland with 229 people aboard when a fire in the cockpit raged out of control and the plane plunged into the Atlantic five miles off the coast of Nova Scotia. Lauren traveled to the crash scene to report on the crash. She spoke with officials and victim's family members there while Sylvia remained in New York, gathering information from sources in the States. When John Kennedy Jr.'s plane went down in July 1999, Sylvia was in Bermuda on maternity leave. Lauren was the only person who knew exactly where Sylvia was, and Lauren had promised not to tell anyone where she was, no matter what. Lauren kept her promise and worked the story with Sylvia. This tragedy was soon followed by the crash of EgyptAir Flight 990 on October 31, 1999. The Boeing 767 departed Los Angeles for Egypt, with a stopover in New York. Shortly after leaving Kennedy, it nosedived into the Atlantic Ocean about sixty miles south of Nantucket Island, off the coast of Massachusetts. The cause of the crash that killed the 217 people aboard was believed to be a deliberate act by one of the pilots who steered the plane into the ocean intentionally, though this accepted theory could not be proven.

Naturally, Lauren and Sylvia worked together after the 9/11 terrorist attacks. The attacks brought everyone closer together. Lauren's and Sylvia's cubicles in the newsroom had been a row apart, but after the World Trade Center was destroyed, for convenience Lauren took the space next to Sylvia that had recently been vacated. The very first 9/11 story they worked on together was to talk with a number of other pilots who told them, to a man, that the airlines' pilots could not have been at the controls, because no pilot would have flown an aircraft into those buildings, even if guns were held to their heads.

That unprecedented act of terrorism changed the worldview for many Americans and altered the way New Yorkers lived their lives. Like everyone else who had loved ones living or working in Manhattan at that time, we immediately reached for the phone and couldn't get through. Ginny was at work and called Lauren's apartment and then tried to reach her at work while I kept trying her cell phone. She lived a safe-enough distance away from the World Trade Center and her office was in Long Island, but her job as a reporter took her all over the city, and we had no idea where she was that morning.

Finally, Lauren picked up. Seeing it was me calling from my cell phone, the first thing she said was, "I'm okay, Dad. I'm in Long Island." I could tell Lauren was busy and I knew she had a lot of work to do. She was safe, and that was all that mattered. I told her to be careful and called Ginny to tell her Lauren was okay.

News about the September 11 attacks was still unfolding when we got off the phone with Lauren. I knew she had a job to do and that there was a potential for danger whenever she walked out the door, that day more than ever. But she wasn't going to stop doing her job, and I wouldn't have wanted her to stop doing it. That was part of what made Lauren who she was.

Then, just two months later, on November 12, 2001, American Airlines Flight 587 to the Dominican Republic crashed in the Belle Harbor neighborhood of Queens just after takeoff from JFK. Lauren and Sylvia jointly covered that crash for *Newsday* as well. It was eventually determined that pilot error during wake turbulence brought down the Airbus A300, which killed 265 people, including five people on the ground.

After working so closely together for so long on such emotional and often tragic stories, Sylvia and Lauren formed a strong bond. Looking back, Sylvia realizes how quickly their relationship developed. She recalls Lauren seeming to want to be friends first, while she remained hesitant. It was something they would laugh about in later years, and when Lauren got sick, she said to Sylvia, "I know you used to think I was annoying, but you love me now, right?"

"Yes," Sylvia acknowledged. "I love you."

5

Lauren traveled extensively in her thirties, and one of the last trips she took was one that I planned with her with the hope of saving her life.

I had never been an advocate for alternative medicine, but following a much too brief period of remission, after which Lauren's cancer returned, I was for anything that might possibly help stop the disease from spreading and make her feel better. When it came to Lauren, I didn't care how these goals were achieved. I would have tried anything or gone anywhere, and I was more than willing to personally give up everything I had for just the slightest hope that it would benefit Lauren. She and I had talked about this topic before, so I knew she was open to other treatment options, too.

Desperate to do something to help her, I read anything and everything I could to find about new and/or unconventional cancer treatments. One that looked particularly promising was something called proton beam therapy.

In this therapy, a particle accelerator is used to target the tumor with a focused beam of protons. Just as with standard radiation treatment, the process of ionization that occurs damages the DNA of cells, ultimately killing them. Cancerous cells, because of their high rate of division and their reduced ability to repair damaged DNA, are particularly vulnerable to attack on their DNA.

It sounded complicated at first, but it made sense after a while, especially when I learned that standard X-ray therapy as well as proton beam therapy work on the principle of selective cell destruction.

The major advantage of proton treatment over conventional radiation, however, is that the energy distribution of protons can be much more tightly focused on tumor cells without affecting surrounding, healthy cells.

Proton treatment can be quite effective, but perhaps its most significant drawback is its cost and the fact that most health insurers will not cover it; proton beam therapy is an out-of-pocket expense which is too financially burdensome for most patients.

In January 2007, I convinced Lauren to fly with me to the University of Texas MD Anderson Cancer Center in Houston to learn more about the treatment. We stayed overnight and met with several oncologists who sold their treatment as one that could potentially save Lauren's life, but they gave it to us straight, telling us that there was no guarantee of success and that Lauren would have to temporarily relocate to Texas for the treatment.

On the flight back to Boston, Lauren seemed cautiously optimistic. Ultimately, her hesitation about participating in the proton beam therapy program stemmed from the fear of having to endure side effects similar to those she experienced during the chemotherapy and radiation treatments she had gone through over the past two years. At least that's what she told us was her reason for ultimately backing out of the risky treatment option at the last minute.

However, we didn't know that there was a conflict Lauren was facing at home as well as inside her body. We later learned from one of Lauren's closest friends that her husband of less than a year (her second husband) had made it clear to her that he was against her seeking alternative medical treatments.

"You can either go it alone, or we can do this together," Al told Lauren. "If we did pursue the treatment, how much are we going to spend from the 401K? Twenty thousand? Thirty thousand? The whole amount in there? And what about me? I am going to be broke. Am I going to be in debt for the next thirty years?"

Lauren never revealed any such conflict to us. She was scared, but she kept this to herself in order to spare us any further despair about her terminal situation. She was trying to be considerate to the very end, and it was only after Lauren died that I found out about this as well as a lot of other things that my daughter went through in her final days.

After Lauren's passing, I was very grateful that her friends had confided in me, sharing their thoughts and memories of Lauren, which I never would have known otherwise. I am still finding out new bits of information about her to this day and experiencing them for the first time. In some way, it feels like Lauren is still alive as I discover these things about her that I did not know previously.

Her friend Eden Laikin recalled one of the last visits she made to Lauren's apartment and the additional stress she witnessed firsthand. Ginny and Al were there together, and Eden immediately sensed that there was a lot of tension between them. Lauren was in her bedroom, clearly wanting to separate herself from all the animosity in the apartment as the people closest to her tried to find a way to deal with her dying.

The instant Lauren heard Eden's voice, she yelled through the door for her friend to come inside. Eden saw Lauren sitting up in bed, her legs, feet, and stomach swollen. It had become difficult for her to walk, and Eden knew her friend's body was shutting down. Lauren told Eden that her family was arguing about her traveling to seek out doctors who offered radical treatments that might help her. She confided to Eden that she just wished all the arguing would stop. Eden lay down on the bed next to her dying friend and tried to help Lauren breathe slowly and to meditate, to just be still and try to block out everything else.

Eden remembered that Lauren did calm down and feel better. Then Lauren took out her laptop and, right in front of Eden, started writing what would be one of her last "Life, with Cancer" columns. It was the one in which she revealed to her readers that she had two months to live.

Eden watched Lauren's slow, deliberate keystrokes on the keyboard until she completed the column. Lauren then turned the screen toward Eden for her to read what she had written. But before she allowed Eden to read, she made her promise not to reveal to Ginny and me any of what she was about to read. Eden gave her word, and then put a hand to her mouth in awe of what she read. Lauren wrote about how it felt to be given a death sentence, to know pretty precisely when you were going to die. When she finished the article, Eden looked at Lauren and without saying anything, embraced her in an extended hug.

We wanted her to pack her bags to visit doctors who might save her life, but she was preparing herself for life's final journey and trying to make peace with that.

Four

What Cancer Gives: Anger, Not Wisdom

"Live each day as if it is your last."

Nope. Can't do it.

While sometimes I am the carpe diem sort of girl, I want to live each day like just another day. I want to watch "When Harry Met Sally" for the 17th time or surf the Internet for new pictures of Britney Spears' bald head. Then I want to cap it off by several hours of reading. Forget Tolstoy, though. I'd rather read People *magazine. Why do I have to cram life into 20 seconds, while other people have the luxury of doing it over the span of 20 years?*

"Hell, no," says a friend of mine about the "live each day" mantra. She just turned 36 and goes for chemotherapy regimens every three weeks for the foreseeable future. Some weekends she just wants to be lazy and sleep until noon and not worry she is squandering precious time.

"You are so brave."

No, I'm not.

Firefighters and police officers who plunge head first into dangerous situations are brave. A child protective worker who gets paid next to nothing and tries to be a mother to as many as 50 dysfunctional families is brave. Those people chose their positions in life. Cancer chose me. It's not bravery that gets me up every morning to try to beat back the monster. It's a survival instinct that kicks in, pure Darwinism.

The fact is, most of the time I am scared to death. I wear Band-Aids far too long because I can't take the agony of pulling them off. I hate needles (though I don't know anyone who likes them). Why is it that people who hate getting blood drawn are the ones who usually end up with serious illnesses that require getting stuck often? It's a mystery of the universe, much like why tornadoes seem to seek out trailer parks to do their damage.

From *Newsday*, "Life, with Cancer," March 6, 2007,
"What Cancer Gives: Anger, Not Wisdom" by Lauren Terrazzano

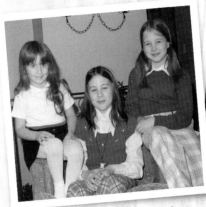

"LT" at age 4 with friends Judy and Katy Greer
© Frank Terrazzano

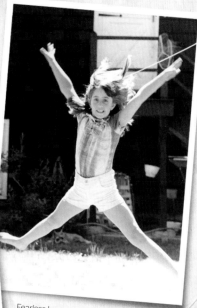

Fearless Lauren practicing for Pop Warner
cheerleading, age 6
© Frank Terrazzano

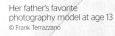

Her father's favorite
photography model at age 13
© Frank Terrazzano

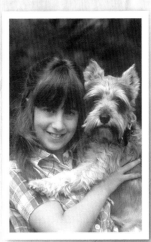

Lauren at age 10 with Benji, who was
often dressed in doll clothes
© Frank Terrazzano

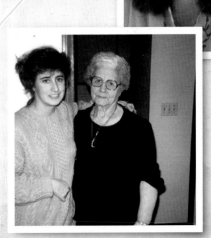

Lauren at age 20 with her Nona Grace,
just before leaving BU to study in Rome
for spring semester
© Frank Terrazzano

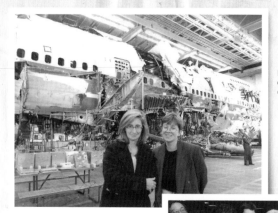

Lauren and Sylvia Adcock in front
of the remnants of TWA flight 800
© 2000, Newsday LLC

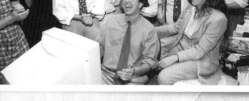

Newsday staff at the announcement of their Pulitzer Prize win in
April 1997; Lauren and Sylvia Adcock are in the center
© 1997, Newsday LLC

Monica Quintanilla and Lauren in 1998 during their
hike in the Tetons
© Monica Quintanilla

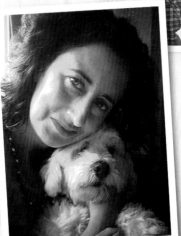

Lauren and Bart
© Frank Terrazzano

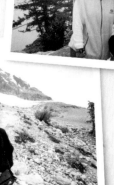

In Canada, 1998
© Peter Gabriele

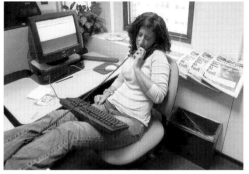

Back to work at the *Newsday* office after surgery, 2005
© Monica Quintanilla

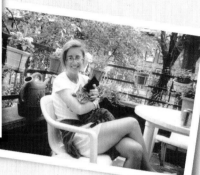

Lauren with her cats in her first apartment on the West Side, 2000
© Frank Terrazzano

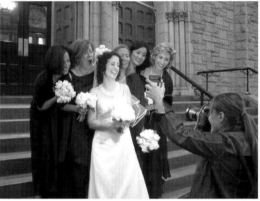

Lauren and her "de facto siblings," from left: Dina Fernandez, Sylvia Adcock, Lauren, Monica Quintanilla, Tomoeh Murakami Tse, and Leah Ritchie
© Archie Tse

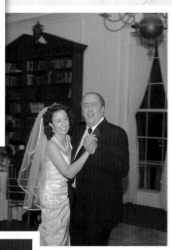

Lauren and her father, Frank
© Archie Tse

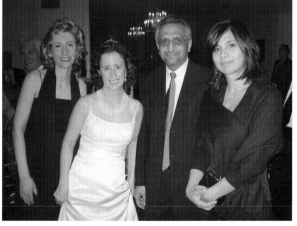

Leah Ritchie and Lauren with Dr. Ashfaq and Mrs. Ashfaq
© Archie Tse

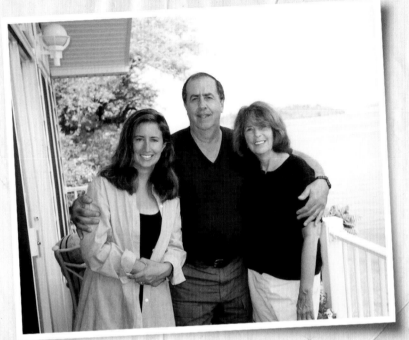

Lauren, her dad Frank, and her mom Ginny in 2002
© Frank Terrazzano

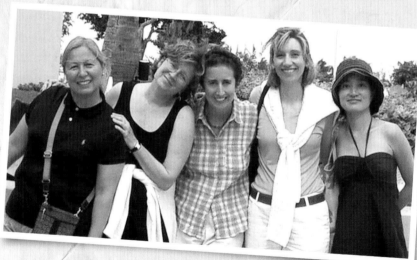

Monica Quintanilla, Sylvia Adcock, Lauren, Leah Ritchie, and
Tomoeh Murakami Tse in the Bahamas, 2005
© Archie Tse

1

W hen she was growing up, Lauren was never far from a Nancy Drew mystery novel. Somewhere around the fifth grade she became hooked on the stories of the fictitious young heroine who solved mysteries and crimes with her guile and her independent spirit. Once Lauren discovered this series of books, she would take them with her everywhere. And on Sundays, when she went with us to visit her grandmother, she was sure to have a book or two with her. By the end of the day she would be curled up in a chair and reading for hours. She loved it. She could have written for the series herself if that had been the direction she chose to take with her writing, but journalism was her calling. When she had a chance to write a bit of an investigative piece of her own about the books she loved so much as a young girl, she jumped at the opportunity. The article she wrote appeared in *Newsday* on November 18, 1998. We saw how excited she was while she was working on it, and doubly so after the article appeared in the paper. She looked just like she did when she was a kid and in the middle of a Nancy Drew mystery that was just getting to the good part.

The name Mildred Augustine Wirt Benson might not mean anything to most people, but to Lauren she was a major celebrity and a female role model, someone who Lauren admired once as a captivated ten- to fifteen-year-old and still as a thirty-year-old writer herself. Benson was the creator of the characterizations (if not the original characters) in the Nancy Drew series and had ghostwritten the first twenty-three Nancy Drew books. "Carolyn Keene" was the pseudonym that Benson and all other Nancy Drew ghostwriters have written under. The first Nancy Drew book Benson penned was released in 1930. In 1998, Lauren was delighted to find that Benson was alive. She was ninety-three and living in Toledo, Ohio.

The Benson piece originated after Lauren noticed the release of a new book that set out to explore the enduring popular-culture appeal of the Nancy Drew and Hardy Boys mystery series. Initially, Lauren sought the authors of this book to interview for her article.

"For me," Lauren wrote, "Nancy simply represented being independent and strong and quietly confident during a time when teen heroines routinely were not. While other girls were wasting hours in the mirror or fawning over adolescent crushes, Nancy was more interested in solving mysteries. Locked in a broom closet, poisoned or struggling to free herself from a cobwebbed cellar, she always used her smarts to triumph in the end."

But the purpose of the article wasn't just about paying homage to the fictitious girl sleuth that had given her so much joy to read about as a youth. Lauren had a personal mystery of her own she wanted to unravel.

She wrote, "I was bemused that academics and students of pop culture were still trying to understand how Nancy Drew managed to tiptoe into the consciousness of so many women. What did she have that makes my own mother save my books in a cardboard box in the garage, hoping to pass them on someday to a future granddaughter? And why is it that so many of my friends and colleagues confess to having read the mysteries?

"Nearly two decades after I first read them, I set out to find out who and what was behind these books that so influenced my childhood."

After speaking with the authors of the book *The Mysterious Case of Nancy Drew and the Hardy Boys,* she still wanted more answers, so she decided to go directly to the source.

Mildred Augustine Wirt Benson.

Lauren contacted her by phone for an interview, and Benson agreed. Lauren learned that, like herself, Benson had worked as a journalist. In fact, the number she dialed was the newsroom of a Toledo, Ohio, newspaper where Benson was still working and writing. She wrote a feature column titled "On the Go with Millie Benson," which advised and informed older citizens on various topics of interest. Benson had been with the paper for fifty-five years.

Lauren had done her research on the original Nancy Drew novelist, and she was amazed not only by everything Benson had accomplished as a female author of her generation, but also by how active she still was as a writer. Lauren discovered that Benson earned a master's degree from the prestigious University of Iowa School of Journalism in 1927, and in doing so broke new ground by becoming the first woman to successfully complete Iowa's advanced level of study.

There was much to admire about this woman who, after attaining her degree, had ventured to New York City to look for a position as a journalist. She interviewed with a number of prominent publishers, but did not receive an offer at first.

Lauren saw a strong parallel between Benson's professional path as a journalist and her own, and she was proud to have even this most modest literary connection to the iconic author.

In the interview, Lauren learned that soon after returning to Iowa, Benson had received a phone call from the Stratemeyer Syndicate, one of the publishers she had interviewed with in New York. The syndicate was a successful producer of mystery and adventure serial books for children. They offered Benson $125 a week to create the first of a couple dozen Nancy Drew mysteries. She was required to sign away all rights to the characters, but she jumped at the opportunity, and the writing she produced would change her life and affect the lives of millions of teenage girls for generations.

Lauren also learned that in the early 1980s the Nancy Drew series publisher revised Benson's early books because of complaints about the portrayal in them of immigrants as ignorant and about blacks in the stories being frequently suspected in crimes. These politically correct versions of Benson's original works were the ones that Lauren had read, and Benson, no bigot or racist by any stretch, had been highly critical of the changes. Benson believed that in the revision process, key aspects of Nancy Drew's character were bastardized and that her instinctive nature and gumption were refined to the point of banality. Lauren read several original letters that Benson had written to Stratemeyer Publishing expressing her opinion about the revisions to the early stories.

In speaking with Benson herself, however, Lauren found, to her dismay, that the groundbreaking author had little to say about Nancy Drew, who some literary scholars have touted as an early iconic feminist character. Perhaps Benson was too far removed by then from the characters she had helped develop some seventy years earlier. In the end, while Lauren may not have solved the mystery of where the fictitious Nancy Drew came from—her search generated more questions than it turned up answers—it had been a genuine thrill and an honor for Lauren to meet the woman who was responsible for bringing to life so many mystery stories in the Nancy Drew series.

Mildred Augustine Wirt Benson, the original "Carolyn Keene," died four years after the interview she gave to Lauren.

When Lauren asked the author about the genesis of the character of Nancy Drew, Benson replied, "Nancy was far ahead of her time as an independent character. But," she said poignantly, "I made her as girls *wished* they were, not as they were."

Lauren had always wished she could be like Nancy Drew, but in a lot of ways she *had* been like her. As she continued to grow as a journalist, she began to further assert with editors her desire to cover social and welfare issues on Long Island. She became a social sleuth of sorts, a journalistic Nancy Drew, looking for answers to societal problems, especially those involving the care and welfare of children, the elderly, and other less fortunate members of our society who had been neglected or otherwise dismissed. It was a mystery to her how certain social problems could be allowed to continue unchecked.

I had always told Lauren, "Don't be afraid to ask questions." For most of my life, I was very introverted. That's how I was when I started working at Louise's Ravioli. But very quickly I learned from the owner of the company—a super salesman and an entrepreneur—that you either spoke up or you got walked all over. It was a lesson that changed me from an introvert to very outgoing. I thought this was an important lesson for my daughter as well. I would tell Lauren this story and say, "So don't be afraid to ask questions." And she wasn't, despite having to ask some very difficult ones.

Lauren perhaps wrote most often, if not most passionately, about child abuse cases. There were many horrible stories of mistreatment, from neglect and emotional abuse to acts of physical violence and sexual molestation, actions that were perpetrated both in state and private care facilities as well as in the children's own homes. Some of those children died as a result of the injuries inflicted upon them. It sickened Ginny and me to hear about those incidences and the frequency with which they occurred. Lauren was greatly bothered as well, but that was precisely why she wrote about those issues. To not acknowledge the problems or pretend they didn't happen would have made her feel worse. She believed that uncovering and expos-ing difficult issues was a key element in eliminating abuse, mistreat-ment, and other forms of social exploitation.

2

In the organized chaos that was Lauren's workstation at *Newsday* was an array of humorous cartoons and inspirational quotes. They would evolve over time, removed and replaced by those more timely or more relevant to what she currently was going through. One that was always there was a tattered and taped-together maga-zine ad that read: "THE PEOPLE WHO ARE CRAZY ENOUGH TO THINK THEY CAN CHANGE THE WORLD ARE THE ONES WHO DO." It was from the old Apple computer "Think Different" slogan. She may have kept it there to remind herself that one per-son really can make a difference, as did Steve Jobs, the cofounder of Apple, who changed many people's vision of the world.

Lauren often discussed with us her desire to write about and expose the shortcomings of our society. She was passionate in her belief that by writing about topics such as the homeless problem and child and elderly abuse, the politicians would take notice and do something about it.

Sometimes a lot of little things can add up to make a big difference, one person at a time, one story at a time. When Lauren began to see where there was a real need for civic and social change in the Long Island community she was covering, she dove headlong into the problem. She got personally involved so that she could write about the topic with more knowledge and empathy, which then made it easier for her to convey the full emotions of the story to her readers.

Jessica Kowal, who Lauren knew from graduate school at Columbia, had been with *Newsday* about a year before Lauren came aboard. They grew closer during the couple of years they were both working out of the Long Island office, before Jessica moved to the Queens desk. They covered different areas of suburban Long Island, which is generally considered to be a massive expanse of idyllic middle- and upper-class families. Lauren saw Long Island differently.

Because it is located outside the hustle and bustle of the city but close enough to commute easily into Manhattan and the other boroughs, many people falsely believe that you magically leave crime and poverty behind once you cross over into Nassau County or Suffolk County. But there are problems even in the best neighborhoods, as well as pockets of poverty and depressed areas occupied by people whose daily lives are plagued by social, health, and welfare hardships.

The landscape of Long Island can be deceptive in that sense. With its broad, tree-lined streets, expensive beachfront homes, and good schools, far removed from the more conspicuous dangers and visible inner-city blight that can be found in and around the New York metropolitan area, there is a false sense of security.

Lauren recognized this. She did not want to turn a blind eye to problems but to tell the stories of forgotten people who lived in these less visible neighborhoods. The poor; individuals who were going through hard times; concerns involving various social institutions; mental health care; and the juvenile justice system were some of the areas of concern that Lauren was interested in writing about. At one point, she approached her editors and argued fervently that this should be her beat at the paper. Initially, the powers that be rebuffed her suggestion. It was a hard sell since it wasn't a typical beat. Lauren was asking for a lot more than she perhaps realized, but she was committed to pursuing social services stories, which boiled down to how federal, state, and local governments and municipalities helped, or failed to help, individual people in need in Long Island communities. She would continue to go out and find these kinds of stories, taking her responsibility as a journalist to a new level in the process.

One weekend Lauren went up to the Hamptons, the popular seaside resort community along the eastern tip of Long Island where the wealthy go to vacation and party. However, she did not go there to interview the beautiful people and celebrities; she ended up spending the entire time with a homeless family to find out how children with working parents could be without a home and to experience what their daily life was like.

It was early 2000, a time when homeless cases were on the rise all around Suffolk County. Lauren wanted to get to know some of the people who were without permanent homes and provide a first-hand account of how they lived, sacrificed, and survived each day together. She hoped to change the perception that many people had of what a homeless person looked like; the stereotypical image of a disheveled man in ragged clothes who was talking to himself while pushing around a shopping cart with all his belongings inside was not close to the truth of what Lauren saw. More often than not, it was a young person or even a child in a family where both parents worked. The reality was especially troubling and much sadder than the image of the Depression-era hobo. Lauren wanted to make this clear by writing about the subject intimately, so she spent a weekend with a family of ten who shared two motel rooms. She ate meals with them and took the long bus rides to school with the children. She got to know them well.

The family initially lost their home when their landlord evicted them. Because they were such a large family, finding affordable housing was difficult. They sought housing help from the Department of Social Services, which placed them in a succession of shelters and motels.

Lauren's story focused on seventeen-year-old high-school senior Louis Daniels, the oldest of eight siblings who ranged from ages four to fourteen and were cared for by their mother and Louis's stepdad, a warehouse worker. Against this ever-distracting backdrop of being homeless, Louis quietly pursued academic excellence, becoming a high-ranking honors student and earning a full academic scholarship to Yale University.

"Homeless off and on since the fourth grade," Lauren wrote, "he would tell his friends to send mail to his grandmother's house in Deer Park, New York, embarrassed that they might find out. He never told teachers about his situation, reluctant to invoke pity or special treatment."

Louis told Lauren, "It forced me to be sensitive about other people's situations and forced me to be grateful about anything that happens," he said. "I don't take things for granted. I know you can lose 'em really fast."

Louis said he had been blessed with the ability to focus on academics even though he shares two adjoining motel rooms with his seven siblings.

"I don't let things distract me that easily," he said, adding that when things got really noisy, he would walk a half-hour to the local library to study.

When the county placed Louis's family at a motel in Southampton, he would take the 5:15 AM county bus for the nearly two-hour one-way ride to his school. He rode with his younger brothers who attended a nearby elementary school. After his last class, he would wait for them to get out so he could travel home with them. He also worked the drive-through window at a Wendy's restaurant for twenty-four hours a week.

Louis applied to several schools, including Harvard University, where he was wait-listed, before accepting the scholarship to Yale.

Lauren's story about Louis and his family was one of inspiration and hope, and it ended up being the graduation story that spring in *Newsday*.

With stories like that, Lauren's editors finally relented and agreed that she could have the community beat. However, it was with the stipulation that in the end she deliver something more than just a sob story. They wanted her to go further—for example, to expose institutional problems and show how they could ultimately be solved, or to reveal how state government and its policies negatively impact the broader community. They wanted her to explain how laws could be changed. By reaching beyond the individual "human interest" story and focusing on social service issues to see what was lacking and what could be done to improve people's lives, the newspaper could then make a real difference; and having a beat writer working those stories would be justifiable. Lauren understood this. By looking at the bigger picture, she knew that she would be able to reach more people and have a greater impact on readers. She took this approach and ran with it.

Jessica Kowal was among a number of journalists at *Newsday*, many of them Lauren's friends, who were looking to move away from *Newsday* and get on at larger papers or be relocated to the paper's Queen's office. Many of them did, in fact, move on, but Lauren stayed where she was. Some of her colleagues did not fully understand this. One of them was Jessica, who had encouraged Lauren to join her and work downtown. There were major advantages to working in the city, the least of which was the elimination of a daily commute to Long Island. The real benefit was the bigger canvas that was New York. The larger playing field, Jessica pointed out, would allow a social journalist like Lauren to showcase her skills and have an impact on the lives of millions of people living and working in the city. But Lauren would have none of it. She remained committed to what she was doing with the social services stories on Long Island.

I was aware of Lauren's decision. I had always told her that she could ask my advice on anything, but ultimately she had to do what was best for her, and her alone.

One thing that Jessica did understand was that Lauren was by no means sacrificing ambition for integrity. She knew Lauren to be extremely competitive, as much so as any journalist she had ever known. Lauren would get quite upset if another paper beat her to publication of a story she was working on. She always thought all the stories she wrote deserved to be on the front page, and she would be disappointed if they were not, but this was not because she wanted to have her name in the byline. What compelled her was her desire to have the story recognized for what it was. She worked long and hard on her stories because she felt they were important, so if they did not get the attention they deserved, the injustice or problem she wrote about would, she believed, continue to be overlooked. This was the kind of achievement that drove her: the impact her story had on people and a community and the potential it had to enlighten opinion and elicit change for the better.

For Jessica, there was one story that perfectly epitomized how Lauren used her craft as a journalist to promote the greater good. It may not have been one of the more trumpeted or far-reaching social welfare stories she did, but it clearly exemplified how she was able to utilize her journalism as an instrument of reform and a means to an end.

The story involved a local minister who stole thousands of dollars in charity funds designated for poor families and children and used the money to purchase a number of expensive cars for herself, including several new Mercedes-Benzes. Lauren's investigative work revealed the minister's misappropriation of the funds, and the story, when it broke, generated quite a stir. But what thrilled Lauren was the police investigation that the story prompted and the subsequent arrest of the minister. By working hard and exposing the minister's misdeeds, Lauren was rewarded with a genuine sense of accomplishment. This made Lauren want to continue doing what she was doing on Long Island.

Lauren was able to churn out many stories like this one because of her ability to develop sources in social services. These were people who, like she, cared about the collective problems of individuals in a community and wanted to see things improved. In many cases, the whistleblowers who talked to Lauren in secret were risking their livelihoods. She earned their trust and they confided in her on sensitive issues that could—and often did—cause real trouble for the various agencies they represented. At her desk in the newsroom, Lauren would often be seen speaking quietly into the phone as she worked her sources and developed her stories. Other reporters were sometimes loud and you could hear everything they were saying, but not Lauren. Although she was very outgoing and had lots of friends, she was a very private person in many ways, and this was one of them. She was intense, and when she was working it was as if nothing else was going on around her as she focused on what she was doing.

Another example of a typical Lauren Terrazzano story that Jessica shared with me resulted from a trip Lauren made to the state capital of Albany. It was during the years that she and Lauren worked out of the Long Island office together. Instead of coming back with a story about the governor or some other political figure or event, Lauren had written a story about the state's elimination of college programs for inmates at a women's prison. Helping uncover the truth behind the eliminations and speaking for people who didn't have a voice or enough influence to be heard were exactly the kinds of things that got Lauren fired up, fueled her ambition, and made her such a force as a journalist.

3

While Lauren was at Tewksbury High School she wrote for the school paper, *Smoke Signals,* and she was also in the International Club. During the summers of her junior and senior years she interned with a local newspaper, the *Wilmington Town Crier.* The paper awarded her a $500 scholarship to help her pursue her career in journalism, which would begin with school that fall at Boston University. During her senior year, Lauren had applied to and was accepted at a number of universities. Ginny and I accompanied her to all of the open houses, whether they were local or out of state, but in the end there was really no choice for Lauren—Boston University had always been her school of choice. Probably from the time she was twelve years old, whenever anybody would ask her where she wanted to go to college, she would always tell them Boston University, and, from the day she received her acceptance letter from the school until the first day of classes in the fall semester, she talked about it incessantly.

For a middle-class working family like ours, the tuition expenses were quite high, but fortunately the equity in our home enabled us to provide the funds necessary to send Lauren to her school of first choice. Lauren had given more than a little consideration to the possibility of commuting to school from Tewksbury while living at home, partly to save money on living expenses, but it was something that I greatly discouraged. The ride into city each day would not have been too serious a burden—a half-hour drive down I-93 South—but I thought it would be in her best interest to live at school. A lot of her friends were going much farther away, so this would be a once-in-a-lifetime experience for her. Living at home would afford her little opportunity to make friends at school, so the extra money for room and board would be money well spent. That's the way I saw it, and that was what Lauren did.

I learned much about Lauren's private feelings, concerns, and insecurities around the transition to BU many years later, after her death, when I read the diary she kept during college.

Like her graduation day would be four years later, the weather on her first day at Boston University was raw and drizzly. The conditions also seemed to dampen her spirits. Upon taking her first steps onto the grounds of the expansive campus, Lauren experienced a conflicting range of emotions, one minute feeling euphoria about the new and wonderful experiences that lay ahead and the next minute feeling scared, confused, and alone.

Away from home for the first time, Lauren immediately felt the symptoms of homesickness. She missed her family, her friends from high school, and everything that was familiar and had meaning in her life. As time went by, she felt that she did not belong at BU, that she did not fit in. She was not making friends as easily as she had hoped, and most of the other students appeared distant, elusive, and indifferent. A contributing factor to her feelings of isolation was the fact that the school had to put her up temporarily at a local Sheraton Hotel because the dormitories were all full when she arrived. She felt like a friendless, faceless ghost wandering the campus by day, and at night a social outcast who was not permitted to interact with the student body.

At the end of the first week, feeling completely alienated, she called home, crying, and asked to be picked up and taken home. I was still at work, so she had to wait until the end of the day. In the meantime, she decided to get started on a class assignment and stopped by the Isabella Stewart Gardner Museum, off campus along the southern edge of the Back Bay Fens, to begin her research. There, she met a classmate who was working on the same assignment. His name was David, and he was from England. They finished what they had to do and then went for tea together at a nearby café. Their conversation drifted toward the dilemma Lauren was experiencing. David's views about adversity and strength and enduring the hardships life throws one's way convinced her not to leave—at least not yet. The young Englishman helped her to recognize that there was an adjustment period involved that she had to get through. She still worried that she would not make a single friend, but she became determined not to give up and go back home defeated. When she got back to her room she called home and told her mom to forget what they talked about earlier: she was staying.

When I spoke to Lauren later, I reassured her that she was doing the right thing. I knew this from my own experiences; I suffered the same insecurities. I told her that as time went on all would change for the better. I told her I had gotten through it, and so would she.

Lauren was well aware that being an only child had its advantages, but there were inherent burdens as well. As she wrote in her diary, she believed that up until this time she had lived a somewhat sheltered life, which only exacerbated the difficult time she was having adjusting to her new environment. The temptation to just run back home was always there, but she fought it, not wanting her weakness to get the better of her and keep her from achieving her goals. She had worked hard throughout high school, putting just about all of her time and effort into her studies so she could get good grades and put herself in the best possible position to be accepted into Boston University and study journalism. Now that she had gotten this far, she did not want to throw it all away. Her biggest fear was failing, flunking out, and ruining all the plans she had for herself.

Lauren made it through the first week at BU, but meeting new people continued to be difficult for her. She actually started to think that she might be okay with it. She had always been an open and trusting person who enjoyed meeting different people and making friends, but if this was how things were in the real world, she told herself, then she would just have to acclimate herself to it. Living out of a hotel made it easier and cheaper to visit a nearby fast-food restaurant for meals. Late one afternoon she went to get something to eat and sat down alone, something she never thought she would do. To her surprise, a feeling of independence washed over her and she found the experience to be quite liberating. However, when she ran into a couple of former high school classmates at the restaurant the following day, she became aware of just how lonely she still was. On top of that, the workload was increasing. The amount of reading she had to do, the homework, studying, all the projects and assignments—it was overwhelming. Even if she had had friends, she wondered how she would find the time to socialize with them.

Lauren made her mother and me aware of these concerns. I knew she was just looking for a shoulder to cry on, and a little reassurance seemed to do the trick. Coming home for the weekend after her first two weeks of school was just what she needed. She was so glad to be back in the comfortable and familiar environment she knew so well and sleeping in her own bed. She had the best night's sleep she had had since she left, not having to worry about class schedules, meals, or anything else. Playing with her dog in the backyard brought back fond memories of a childhood that she was barely removed from. She had on occasion in the past criticized her mother's cooking, but she told us it suddenly it tasted better than she had ever remembered. She did not want to leave the security of home, but when the weekend was over she went back to Boston and the Sheraton Hotel.

Later that third week of the semester, Lauren was finally given a room assignment. She found out that she would be in the Towers, on the seventh floor of the dormitory known as the International Floor. Besides the larger concentration of foreign students on the floor, there were also undergraduates studying foreign language or cultures who, by design, all wanted to live together, which Lauren thought would be perfect for her. She also learned that her roommate's name was Hilary.

It was another exciting yet frightening moment for Lauren. She began to think that perhaps she had been an only child for so long that she wouldn't know how to adjust to living with a stranger. She didn't know what her roommate would be like or how they would get along. They might not even like each other.

Lauren could not help calling home, crying. She felt like she had when she was a little girl running to her mother after skinning her knee in the backyard. It was ironic that she once thought that going off to college and living on her own would make her more self-reliant and independent, when now she seemed to be depending on her mother and me more than ever, calling us on the phone crying and complaining all the time, wanting to come home one moment and then changing her mind the next. She recognized that when she had been home during high school she did not talk with us nearly as much as she did the first month she was away at college.

Lauren's roommate and the other girls in her dormitory made her feel insecure from the start. She felt that she did not fit in and that they did not consider her one of them. Deep down inside she believed that she was not like them, and she could not blame them for not liking her. They all appeared more secure and independent than her, which made her feel inferior and unworthy. She just didn't feel accepted. She tried hard, wanting her new floormates to like her, but she also needed her privacy. As an only child, it was something she was used to, and she really wanted to get the best grades she could. When her floormates would play the television or radio too loud and she asked them to lower it, making the request made her feel more like an outcast. She did not want to alienate them, but that was what she thought she was doing, and it bothered her a lot.

With Thanksgiving looming, the thought of returning home over the break was a cause of great concern for Lauren. She thought that when she saw her friends from high school over the holiday weekend, they would tell her how many new friends they had made, how much fun they were having at their schools, how popular they were there, and how many boyfriends they had. Lauren was sure of this and she dreaded it, because she had none of that and was not happy at all.

Her persistent melancholia made her feel stigmatized. The day-to-day struggle with her emotions had her convinced that she was not normal. The lack of control she felt scared her.

Lauren experienced a major setback as her midterm exams approached, but it did not happen in the classroom. It began when a dear friend from home came to visit her in Boston. Suzanne was attending Colby College, and when Lauren first saw her friend, she hardly recognized her. So much about her had changed. She had a different look in her eyes, an unrecognizable expression, and a changed demeanor. She didn't dress the same. More disturbing was her attitude. She had developed a drinking habit and now smoked pot. She also treated Lauren with what Lauren felt was a demeaning and condescending manner. The entire night she never stopped complaining about how boring Boston University was and how her school was so much more fun. She cut Lauren down every chance she could, undermining what little self-confidence Lauren may have been starting to develop.

Beyond disappointment, this experience with her friend shook

Lauren to the core. She wondered if such a metamorphosis was what she would have to go through in order to be a happy and successful college student. Lauren began to see this experience as a dividing line between her old secure world with her parents and the real world outside of the safety of home—a line between self-sufficiency and dependence upon her parents. She thought that the only way she could achieve anything was to give up that security completely, and it scared her because it was something she was not willing to do.

The next day Lauren began to question in earnest not only what she was doing at Boston University but also what she was doing with her life. It was probably the lowest point she had reached in the six weeks she had been away, feeling insecure and insignificant in a big city where she just did not belong. It made her feel fragile and weak because she thought she did not possess the strength to overcome these obstacles and do the things that were necessary to make it in the real world. She longed to be home, where she was loved unquestionably and did not have to try to earn anyone's affections. It was becoming clear to her now that she probably never should have left home.

Lauren felt a now-familiar tug to call home asking to be picked up and taken back to her own bedroom, like Dorothy at the end of her dream in *The Wizard of Oz*. If she had had a pair of ruby slippers she would have clicked them already. But she knew that all she had to do was pick up the phone, and I would have brought her back home almost as fast as if she really had ruby slippers on her feet. But she did not make the call. It took all the strength she had to try to hang on a bit longer. Besides, it was already Sunday and the school week would be starting up again soon. It made no sense to go home only to have to turn right back around to get to class on Monday morning. She stayed put, and it proved to be a turning point for Lauren. The confidence she always had in herself and her abilities was pushing slowly to the surface. Her trepidation and feelings of insecurity, which always came in periodic waves, now seemed to be coming less frequently. That alone made it easier for her to endure during this time.

4

D ina Fernandez met Lauren at Columbia University. It was Dina's first time living out of Guatemala and away from her parents. She felt intimidated and lost in such a large city and attending such a prestigious university, but Lauren immediately befriended her and Dina was very appreciative of her kindness.

Dina had gone to a French school, so English wasn't even her second language. Speaking English was so challenging for her that she would often find herself exhausted from the effort of trying to express herself when she was among a group of American students. But Lauren made her feel comfortable. She was always patient and reassuring, and they became good friends very quickly.

Lauren was genuinely interested both in where Dina came from and in that part of the world. She had never been to Central America. Dina gave her new friend an open invitation to come visit her in Guatemala when they finished school, and Lauren promised that she would take her up on that offer.

The two students had many things in common, most noticeably

a similar background in their family upbringing and values. They were not third- or fourth-generation Ivy League students like some of the students attending Columbia, and in fact they were the first women in their families to get a college education. They would joke with each other about how they were the only Catholic girls in the entire school. It was something they took seriously enough, however, because they made an appointment to see the dean and ask him if they could have Good Friday off—only the Jewish holidays were marked on the calendar. It worked, and all Catholic students were excused from class the Friday before Easter.

Lauren and Dina spent a good deal of time together outside of school, meeting for brunch on Sundays and going to the movies whenever they could, usually taking in a foreign film. Dina likes to take credit for being the one who turned Lauren on to foreign cinema, introducing her to Spanish, Latin American, and French cinema in particular.

They remained close after college, even though Dina went back to live in Guatemala. The physical distance was not much of a problem for Lauren, who was adventurous and loved to travel. She visited Dina in Guatemala numerous times. In February 1999, Lauren flew out there by herself.

In Guatemala at that time, the Truth and Reconciliation Commission findings were released. Truth commissions are investigative bodies established to discover and reveal past wrongdoings by a government and to resolve conflict left over from these past events. They are occasionally set up by states emerging from periods of internal unrest, civil war, or dictatorship. South Africa's Truth and

Reconciliation Commission established by President Nelson Mandela following the dismantling of apartheid is considered the model of truth commissions.

The Historical Classification Commission, Guatemala's truth commission that was created at the end of the country's bloody civil war, which was responsible for the deaths of at least two hundred thousand people since the unrest began there in 1962, called for the investigation into numerous human rights violations and atrocities perpetrated by both sides. The goal was to bring everything out into the light, to learn from three decades of mistakes, and to make changes that would move the nation forward. The final report, titled *Guatemala: Memory of Silence,* had just been published that same month, and despite Lauren's desire to visit her friend and to rejuvenate and heal herself on this Central American vacation, as a journalist this was a news story she just could not resist.

As a journalist herself, Dina was acquainted with one of the members of the commission. He had been a good source of Dina's, and Lauren sought him out for an interview. She also paid a visit to a small town in the western highlands to talk to people to further develop her story. From her investigation, she concluded that a certain number of massacres had taken place in that particular village. However, this number conflicted with what had been reported elsewhere, and consequently what was in the final report.

I remember Lauren being very concerned about this discrepancy. She knew it was not unusual that some villages would have their own accounting for their dead and missing, but she was afraid that the editors at her paper's international desk would think she had not done her job adequately. What Lauren wanted more than anything at this point in her career was to become a foreign correspondent, and she did not want to do anything that might hamper her chances of ever being seriously considered for such a post. She stuck with the number her research turned up, however, and no issue was made of it by *Newsday* or anyone else.

Lauren was not the first (or last) reporter to take note of the inconsistencies of these figures, but at that time no one had publically challenged the numbers of people massacred in the commission's report. There was certainly a silent minority that questioned how accurate they could have been, considering how rapidly the commission came to its conclusion. There had been so much that happened over the course of more than three decades of civil war that the findings would only become more disputed in the succeeding years, until today, when there is no way of knowing for sure how many Guatemalans had been killed en masse, murdered, or gone missing during that time.

5

Despite everything that Dina and Lauren had been through together from their days as journalism students at Columbia University right through the years of friendship that followed, and their adventures in Guatemala and traveling to and from Central America to take part in one another's wedding celebrations, the single most amazing memory that Dina has of Lauren was not something that had happened in Guatemala, but rather in the hospital where Lauren was dying. And writing.

Dina was in New York visiting Lauren for what would be the last time. After learning that Lauren's doctors could no longer effectively combat the aggressive spread of the cancer that was ravaging her body and that it was just a matter of time before it claimed her life, Diana booked the next flight out of Guatemala.

Dina had been following Lauren's column, "Life, with Cancer," online, and at the time of her visit Lauren was working on an installment that would appear in the April 17, 2007, edition of *Newsday*. The article focused directly on the issue of the responsibilities of the tobacco companies, in particular how they market their products for consumption by young women. Although Lauren was listed as a nonsmoker by her doctors because she smoked infrequently for only a few years, and her cancer was not attributed to tobacco use, she went to the mat for all women who had lung cancer.

That month Lauren had seen ads for Camel No. 9 cigarettes in various women's magazines such as *Vogue, Cosmopolitan,* and *Glamour.* The attractive packaging of the cigarettes in a chic pink and black box was designed to instantly draw the attention of teen girls who saw the ads in their favorite magazines. The promotional giveaways for Camel No. 9 when the new brand was launched included berry-flavored lip balm, cell phones, purses, jewelry, and wristbands.

To Lauren, it was obvious that the intent behind the R. J. Reynolds Tobacco Company's marketing scheme for Camel No. 9 was to get young girls to buy their product by making smoking seem glamorous and fun and to associate it with things girls already liked.

Dina was amazed by Lauren's resolve. She was putting the story together essentially from her deathbed. She was very sick at that time. Her eyes were sunken, rimmed by dark circles. She was so thin that the bones in her face were pronounced. Her skin was pale, with a greenish hue, and very dry. It was a deathly complexion that was difficult for her friend to look at. In fact, when Dina first walked into the hospital room she thought it was the wrong one. She could hardly recognize Lauren. She wanted to cry, but she managed to keep it together, knowing that tears, sympathy, and pity were things that Lauren did not want.

But standing beside Lauren's hospital bed that day, watching her work, Dina's emotional experience swung to the other end of the spectrum. She felt proud of Lauren and honored to be counted among her friends, fortunate to be with her; and as a journalist she felt inspired, even envious for what Lauren was doing.

To complete her story, Lauren wanted to get a quote she could use from Camel's marketing director, Craig Fishel, the company man who developed the strategy to entice women to smoke what Lauren privately referred to as "Death Potion No. 9." Fishel was evasive, but Lauren was determined to get the interview. She was on the phone constantly, trying to catch him in his office, sometimes waiting on hold for long periods of time, and then being told he had gone into a meeting.

She was literally dying from lung cancer and at the same time attempting to get in touch with a tobacco-company marketing director. She did not have a lot of time left, but it never diminished her drive to write the story she wanted, the story that she thought was important. She followed her high journalism standards by the book, right to the end.

It was not easy to pin this guy down, but as always, Lauren found a way to get the interview. She had many friends, acquaintances, and sources throughout New York, and she employed this vast network of people to get to Fishel, who finally agreed to give her some of his precious time. When he called her back, Dina was one of the people in her hospital room, along with Monica and Ginny, while Lauren was licking a "morphine lollipop."

The painkiller disguised as candy isn't actually morphine but fentanyl, a synthetic narcotic analgesic that is about 80 times more potent than morphine. Fentanyl is available as a small, grape-flavored cone on a plastic stick; it looks like a lollipop. The medication is absorbed through the mucous membranes in the mouth, where it quickly dissolves into the nervous system and is dispersed throughout the body. The dosage can vary, but its strength makes fentanyl highly addictive. The drug is used primarily to treat "breakthrough" cancer pain—a sudden burst of pain that "breaks through" a patient's normal medications for pain—but it is now also being used to treat pain for various other causes in the hospital setting as well as for injured U.S. soldiers on the battlefield.

Lauren's sense of humor, however, could not be anesthetized so easily. Sometimes, when she was up to it, after the nurse would leave her with the pop in her mouth, she was apt to twirl it around her mouth, turn to one of her friends, and proceed to do her best Shirley Temple imitation, singing:

On the mor-phine lol-li-pop
It's a night trip into bed you hop
And dream away
On the morphine lollipop

This particular afternoon, when the Camel executive called, Lauren wasn't feeling very well. Monica had to hold the phone to Lauren's ear because she was too weak to hold it herself. Given the circumstances, Dina could not believe the way she talked to Fishel. She was nothing but professional, straightforward, and assertive, never mean or plaintive. And she never did mention that fact that she was ill herself. She talked to him as if she were calling from a conventional office setting or even from the comfort of her own home, and as though she was healthy, with her whole life still ahead of her. Fishel had no idea. Dina could not help but wonder how he would have felt if he had seen her as she was—the way she looked as she was talking to him from her a hospital bed, with a morphine lollipop between her teeth. Lauren was the best reporter Dina had ever known, and what she witnessed that day only solidified that in her mind.

Five

Young Adults Find
Common Ground

One look at the logo flashing across the top of the Planet Cancer Website says it all.

"We've done drugs Keith Richards has never heard of."

The Web site, planetcancer.org, has existed for several years, and seeks to fill what was once a huge service and support void for young adults with cancer. It's an often forgotten group of people living with cancer who fall into that scary netherworld between pediatrics and geriatrics, "where no one knows whether to give you a lollipop or have a serious talk about your fiber intake," said Heidi

Adams, one of the Website's founders.

Cancer patients between the ages of 15 and 40 make up 7 percent of the overall cancer population in the United States, according to recent data from the National Cancer Institute, and many experts contend that their mental health needs are often not met. The most common cancers among young people are types of leukemia and lymphoma, and melanoma, she said, but testicular, breast and even lung cancer have fast become cancers of a younger generation.

Although there have historically been emotional support systems in place for other age demographics, young adults are facing a whole set of complexities with dating, fertility and sex, for starters. How many dates should you have before you tell a prospective partner that you've been treated for cancer, and, oh yeah, that it might come back? Will you try to have a child after that toxic round of chemotherapy your body has endured? Questions. Questions.

"Cancer is disruptive at any age, but young adulthood is a time of becoming who you are in terms of career, life path and relationships," said Adams, 39, a Ewing's sarcoma survivor and founder of the Houston-based site that receives support from the Lance Armstrong Foundation.

"Cancer comes along and throws a big old wrench into the works."

That's exactly what happened to me. I remember

Life, with Cancer

scanning the waiting room at Memorial Sloan-Kettering,
looking for anyone even close to my age.

—From *Newsday,* "Life, with Cancer," January 23, 2007,
"Young Adults Find Common Ground," by Lauren Terrazzano

1

WHen Lauren was a young girl, about twelve years old, she
started a neighborhood daycare center of sorts. During the
summer, she would take a couple of youngsters over to our house
and play with them for a few hours while their parents went shopping or to a doctor's appointment. Lauren had them running around
in the backyard if it was a nice day, or if it was raining, she took
them into our basement. There were any number of board games
she played with them, plenty of coloring books, and other books she
read to them. It was something she really enjoyed. She even charged
the parents twenty-five cents an hour. It was a bargain. When she got
a little older she started babysitting on her own for a lot of the same
families and children, and for a lot more than a quarter.

So when it came to the social services stories Lauren wrote as an
adult, it was hardly surprising to Ginny and me that the ones that
most troubled her, the ones that she most intimately involved herself with personally as well as a professionally, had to do with children. In cases where there was even the slightest suspicion of abuse
and/or neglect, Lauren was extra motivated to root out the cause
of the trouble and do whatever she could to remove the child from
an unhealthy environment and get him or her into a better, safer

place as soon as possible. As a journalist, the depth of her concern could be reflected in the number of contacts and sources she had developed within the child welfare community. Lauren was highly protective of sources that wished to remain anonymous, and even for those who made their claims public, she always made sure she kept their relationships as private as possible.

Pam Bell was a social worker who worked closely with Lauren. She was one of many in a vast network of individuals around greater Long Island who, like Lauren, worked to protect children from all forms of mistreatment, violence, and exploitation.

After more than two decades working within the child welfare system both in New York City and Long Island, Pam considered herself to be a committed, if sometimes exhausted, social worker for children. Invariably, this heart-wrenching work takes its toll, and very often she felt exasperated and overwhelmed, on the verge of burnout. During the time that Lauren was around, Pam would look to her for hope and inspiration—hope that things really could be changed for the better, and inspiration that what she was doing really was making a difference as a means to that end.

Pam admired the way Lauren went about her job of exposing the problems (and the misdeeds of individuals) in the child welfare system. Lauren was a hero to many in the field because she would succeed in accomplishing what they often could not. Removing abusive and callous administrators, whether they were in state or privately held positions, was not always easy. The power of the press leveled the playing field, and Lauren wielded that power only to the detriment of those who were hurting children in their care. With the strength of her writing, she became the David to a collective Goliath that all social workers face. Pam was amazed by Lauren's enthusiasm and commitment. It reenergized her personally, and she saw how it inspired others as well.

One scathing investigative piece that Lauren wrote involved children as young as ten who were being held in Suffolk County jail cells. It was memorable for Pam not only because of the impact it had on the community in terms of social reform, but it left an indelible, if somewhat facetious, impression on Lauren's colleagues.

The Long Island children that Lauren wrote about were being kept in jails with adults because a proper juvenile facility (where they should have been housed) could not be built. NIMBY (not in my back yard) complaints foiled plans for its construction at every turn. Community after community rallied against having a prison in their neighborhood. Officials had no choice, they said, but to hold the children in town jails with adults, where one of the most overlooked problems was that the young offenders were not getting the proper education that was required by law. When a ten-year-old boy attempted suicide in one of the jails, Lauren wrote about it. Her story created quite a stir, and soon afterward, plans for the construction of a juvenile jail were underway. Lauren's coworkers at *Newsday*, as well as some of those in the criminal justice system and corrections department, would begin to refer to the new children's jail as the Lauren Terrazzano Memorial Jail.

Lauren was never afraid to go after anyone, at any level, if they were responsible or in any way negligent regarding a child's welfare or safety. Some of the stories Pam helped Lauren develop included an exposé of a state facility for special-needs students that was being investigated for a variety of neglect and abuse allegations. The New York Department of Education began looking into facility practices that included excessive and severe punishments for misbehavior, such as the use of restraints and electric-shock treatments.

In another piece, Lauren called to task the efforts of the city's Administration for Children's Services after a seven-year-old girl died at the hands of her stepfather, despite the agency's awareness that the malnourished child was living in a home where there had been repeated allegations that she was beaten regularly, tied to chairs, and sexually abused.

Pam knows that Lauren helped countless children and their families with her writing, but she also helped social workers like herself, inspiring them and motivating them through her example to recommit themselves to their own work. Even though she is gone, Lauren proved to Pam and to others that one person can make a difference, and that even in times of doubt they are not alone.

2

Brian Donovan recognized right away that there was something special about Lauren. For a young journalist she set especially high standards for herself, regardless of the particular story that she was working on. Brian had been with *Newsday* since 1967, and he had seen many reporters come and go. A fair share, he observed, were often satisfied doing a workmanlike job while winding up, for example, with less than all of the information they needed. Lauren, however, always wanted to get it all, 100 percent, even if she had a limited amount of time to put together a story or if it was going to be a 250-worder on a back page. He witnessed it firsthand, as Lauren always pushed for more—more from herself, more from her sources, more from her editors. She would make that extra phone call, take the time to get the proper records—whatever it took. She displayed a genuine zeal and a level of intensity for her work that Brian rarely saw in seasoned journalists.

Her work was always remarkable, but he recalled Lauren being very self-critical and hard on herself. She was not morose by nature, but rather quick to laugh and smile, and able to see humor in most situations. Without exception, every time he or anyone else approached her following a well-received story she had written, she would sigh and explain that she really wanted to go in some other direction with the story but could not make the leap. What she was saying was that she could have done a better job.

As a journalist, Brian understands the reality that once the reporting aspect of a story is complete, the interviews are done, and you sit down to write it, there is bound to be one aspect or another of the story that you wanted to nail down but just could not. Your guts tell you that something more is there, but you are unable to get the evidence you need to get it on the record.

Before Brian retired after more than thirty-five years as a journalist, he had won a number of awards, including a Pulitzer prize for investigative reporting that he shared with another reporter in 1995 for a series of articles on disability-pension fraud by the Long Island Police Department. He also shared a 1970 Pulitzer Prize for Public Service with other *Newsday* journalists. Their collective three-year investigation and exposure of secret land deals in eastern Long Island led to a series of criminal convictions for, discharges of, and resignations from public and political officeholders in the area. Brian was an investigative reporter for much of his time at *Newsday*, sometimes working on the investigative team, sometimes on the national desk, but always doing some form of investigative reporting. So Brian knows a thing or two about what it takes to become a successful investigative reporter. When Lauren joined *Newsday*, she made an immediate impact.

The overall mission of the investigative team is to look into ways in which systems of public interest and welfare are not working properly, whether through political patronage, corruption, or any way in which the good of the few outweigh the good of the many. There was a broad mandate for these types of long, in-depth projects at *Newsday*, which quickly became known for its investigative pieces, and they won multiple Pulitzer prizes through the years. Having a full time investigative team on staff, one of the first in the country, was a source of great pride for the paper. It was an honor to be chosen to the team, and it required experience and a unique skill set.

Working in a separate office with an elite group of journalists was a major advantage. They had access to an enormous reserve of data and research material. This body of information could be used by all reporters, but the material was much more vital to the investigative team's time-consuming, in-depth investigative stories than it was to the daily, breaking-news reports. So there was always a wall, both physical and imagined, separating the investigative team from the other reporters at the paper.

Brian was on *Newsday*'s investigative team in what he refers to as the "golden era" of newspapers. Journalists would be given a year or sometimes more to complete a project if the information that was coming in was good enough, strong enough, and important enough. One story he worked on toward the end of his career at *Newsday* involved the state's very weak standard of care and level of enforcement for day care and how the state's shortcomings were allowing children to be treated badly and sometimes even seriously abused. Working on this story, Brian got a better understanding of Lauren's particular passion for journalism and the public welfare that prompted her to investigate how children are treated. He had always been struck by Lauren's talents as an investigative reporter, even though that was not her official title. It was a mind-set, a way she approached her work, and the stories she wrote about. She was not satisfied with looking at the surface of things. She wanted to find out what was really going on and where the system was failing.

Brian had hoped to be able to work with Lauren on a project before he left, but it was not to be. Lauren's illness made it impossible. They had begun talking about working together on a project that involved looking at all of the state and county agencies that dealt with children's problems, such as family court, child protective services, and social services, to name just a few. They had even spent some time planning how they would team up, who would do what aspects of reporting, and what kind of stories they would focus on, but then Lauren was diagnosed with lung cancer and those plans never went any further. It was too much for Brian to handle by himself, and he honestly did not think that there was anyone else at *Newsday* who had the insight and the passion to see the project through to the end. Sadly, the story was never written. One of the biggest regrets of Brian's life remains that he and Lauren never got the chance to work together on a comprehensive investigation into the state of child welfare throughout greater New York state. It was something they had both been very excited about.

When Lauren got sick, Brian worked diligently to enter her "Life, with Cancer" columns in various journalism awards contests. The articles were so incredibly moving, he didn't know what else to do. He was impressed by the sincerity and honesty of her writing. He put her entries together for her, entering her in every category of competition ranging from Pulitzer-prize level down to local press-club level. He wrote accompanying letters to awards judges on Lauren's behalf and asked colleagues to do the same.

One colleague who submitted a letter of support on Lauren's behalf was *Newsday* editor Anthony Marro, who simply told them that the work Lauren did in her "Life, with Cancer" column speaks for itself. What it doesn't say, he informed them, is that she produced them while in great pain and under unusually courageous circumstances.

Brian knew the arduous conditions under which Lauren continued to write the weekly articles. He had visited her at home and occasionally found her lying in bed when the pain wouldn't allow her to sit at her desk. But she would transcribe her thoughts on the computer or dictate sentences to a friend. She wrote about her own medical setbacks and diminishing prognosis.

Barry Bearak, a former *New York Times* and *Los Angeles Times* reporter, met Lauren while he was an assistant professor at the Columbia University Graduate School of Journalism. Bearak sat through many of Robin Reisig's summer classes the year that Lauren was her adjunct. He was very impressed with Lauren and her shining idealism. He saw right away how dedicated and enthusiastic she was about training young people to be the best reporters that they could be. She was very proud of her students and she exuded a shining enthusiasm that few instructors possessed. Bearak asked Lauren to work as his adjunct the following semester and she accepted. Bearak was a preeminent foreign correspondent. He had won the 2002 Pulitzer Prize for International Reporting for his coverage of poverty and war in Afghanistan, and Lauren aspired to be a foreign correspondent. Barry's letter to the Society of Silurians, one of the oldest and most prestigious journalism organizations in New York City, helped Lauren win their coveted award. She was posthumously honored by the Society of Silurians, receiving top prize in the science/health reporting category for her writing in her "Life, with Cancer" column. In a letter to me, he explained how his own students were inspired by Lauren after he had assigned some of her columns in his class.

3

Dennis Nowak works for the Department of Social Services on Long Island and currently heads up the Suffolk County Family and Children's Service Administration, which is the division of social services that runs child protective services, adult protective services, foster care, and adoption.

Dennis told me that he will never forget the day that Lauren called him out of the blue and introduced herself as a journalist with *Newsday*. It was around the time that she was concluding her work on the TWA Flight 800 crash story. She told Dennis that she had a special interest in social welfare stories and wanted to become the social welfare beat reporter for the newspaper. She said she needed to get to know the work that he did, and he said he was happy to oblige; it was a cause that could only be helped if more people got involved. Lauren asked if they could meet over lunch so she could hear more about the department, get some background information, and then go from there.

Dennis chose a humble diner in Central Islip that he was familiar with. It was quiet and comfortable. An ideal place to chat, he thought.

He explained to Lauren that he had been with DSS since 1987. In 1992, he was working in the commissioner's office when he was assigned to handle the press, and he described for Lauren how it happened. Just after Christmas that year, Katie Beers, a ten-year-old Long Island girl, was kidnapped by a friend of the family and held prisoner for sixteen days in an underground dungeon in Bay Shore, New York, in Suffolk County. Media from all over began swarming the commissioner's office the moment the story broke, drawing huge national attention. He told Lauren how the commissioner handed him the case file and said, "Here, you deal with the press from now on."

Since then, Dennis had developed good relationships with reporters. He came to respect their work just as they respected his and the work that others did in the department. Lauren confided to Dennis that at one time she had been torn between a career in journalism and social work. Though she had not written about the Katie Beers abduction, Lauren had followed the story closely and told him that it was just such instances of exploitation and abuse of children that made her want to get into the social work aspect of reporting.

It was several years later, when Lauren treated him to lunch at a more upscale restaurant, that Dennis realized what she really thought of their lunch in Central Islip.

Lauren commented, "Remember when we first met and you took me to eat at that crappy diner?"

"Well, it was your dime," Dennis said in a feeble attempt to defend his choice of eateries.

"It wasn't *my* money. It was the paper's. We could have eaten anywhere."

After that, it was something they would laugh about whenever Lauren brought it up, which was not infrequently.

Not long after their inaugural lunch, Lauren began to call on Dennis, asking him if he had any stories for her. She wanted to keep her social welfare beat going, she explained to him, and needed stories, or she would be pulled off the beat by the paper to do daily assignments. Due in part to Dennis's efforts, along with those of other social service workers and resources, losing her social welfare beat was one worry Lauren never had to contend with.

She developed such a trusting relationship with Dennis and the department that she was given access to stories that no other reporter landed. They were so confident that Lauren would protect sensitive information that she was actually allowed to ride along with the child protective staff on their field investigations. She was the first reporter that the department of social services ever granted this special privilege.

As it happened, this was a time when homeless cases were in the news and visible everywhere around Suffolk County, so Dennis had no trouble providing Lauren with an endless supply of individuals who were literally on the outside of society looking in. And Lauren jumped headlong into their personal stories in the same way she approached the subjects of any social welfare piece she was working on. She wanted to meet the families and the children. She wanted to get to know them and get a firsthand account of how they lived, suffered, and survived each day together. She ended up changing the very definition of a homeless person for many people who did not know that most often it is a young person, even a child, who does not have a permanent residence. The stereotypical disheveled man or "bum" in ragged clothes, pushing around a shopping cart with all his belongings inside, is not close to the truth of what a homeless person looks like today. The reality is troubling, much sadder, and far more familial than the Depression-era hobo that comes to mind when many people think of someone who lives on the streets. And Lauren wanted to make this clear by writing from their point of view. She rode on school buses with the children who were picked up from area homeless shelters and motels where they were staying.

One of the features Dennis shared with me as he fondly recalled the work Lauren did with the help of the department of social services is the "home makeover" story with the Lutz family of East

Setauket. Unable to have any children of their own, John and Grace Lutz adopted eighteen children over the years including seven with Down Syndrome. But then tragedy struck when both parents passed away. Their daughter Kathleen came home to take care of her younger siblings after it was agreed by the rest of the family that putting the children into a group home or institution was not an option. A second tragedy followed when Kathleen unexpectedly had a grand mal seizure and was diagnosed with inoperable cancer. Her brother John Jr. stepped in to care for Kathleen and his other siblings. With Kathleen's health stabilized, both brother and sister cared for their family.

After all this, the house they were living in began falling apart. Rain poured in through the ceiling and the cesspool overflowed. The house was unlivable and dangerous. If it could not be repaired, all the children would have to be relocated to state institutions for their well-being. Dennis tried to elicit the help of contractors and construction workers to rebuild the house as a charity project, but his plan went nowhere—until he went to Lauren and told her about the situation.

After talking with all the family members, Lauren wrote a beautiful story about the Lutzes that appeared on the front page of *Newsday* on Thanksgiving Day 2002. The response from readers was overwhelming, and more than $200,000 in donations was received for repairs to the house. Contractors spent two to three weeks making repairs and the family was able to remain in their home. It was something Dennis was very proud to be a part of, and he knew Lauren felt the same way.

Dennis later joked with Lauren that their work together on this project was the genesis of ABC's Emmy Award-winning show *Extreme Makeover: Home Edition*, which debuted a year later in December 2003. Dennis truly believes that it was Lauren's story, which was picked up by several major national magazines, that was the inspiration for the program. Dennis also joked with Lauren that Sarah Michelle Gellar, of *Buffy the Vampire Slayer* fame, would be the one to play her if they made a movie about the show and her role in its origins.

In a twist of irony, nine years later, *Extreme Makeover: Home Edition* did select the now forty-year-old Lutz home to modernize and to make much-needed improvements in a 2011 episode of the program.

Still another charitable organization that Lauren involved herself with was a national movement called the Heart Gallery of America, Inc., which sought professional photographers to work with children who were up for adoption, in foster care, or otherwise institutionalized. Photographs would be taken of the children and then displayed in galleries in the hope of matching children with adoptive families. Suffolk County was the first in New York state to get involved with the Heart Gallery, and Lauren's article on the event landed on the front page again, helping enormously to raise awareness about adoption through foster care and to spur the growth of the organization, which continues to thrive today.

Because of all the work Dennis did with adoptive services, Lauren would occasionally ask him if he thought she would be able to adopt a foster child, and he always told her that she would be the best parent the child could ever hope for.

When Dennis found out about Lauren's illness he was devastated. He had recently suffered the loss of his two sisters to ovarian cancer, a disease that had also claimed his mother's life. He knew that it was a form of cancer than ran in his family, but what happened to Lauren—lung cancer—made no sense to him. He knew she had quit smoking, and he tried to recall if he had ever seen her smoke. He did not, but he remembered a snippet of a conversation he had with her. Lauren had been out on an investigation with a child protective worker, and when she returned she said to him, "My God, the work that you people do is so intense, I found myself chain-smoking with the case worker."

Dennis mock-chastised the case worker for this. "What did you do to her?" he asked. "I told you to take it easy on her. Now you have her chain-smoking."

The last time he saw Lauren, her cancer was in remission and she had returned to work. He visited her in the newsroom and when he saw her, her hair now grown back thick and curly, the first thing he said to her was, "Get over here and give me a hug."

4

In the summer of 2004 Brian Donovan introduced Lauren to the Rev. Bernadette Watkins. "Bern," as many people called her, was well known in the community around Huntington on the North Shore of Long island. To many, she was a living saint.

While this Suffolk County town is a predominantly affluent and well-to-do community, Huntington Station is a section on the south end that stands in stark contrast to the prosperity of the rest. Perhaps best known as being the birthplace of Walt Whitman, one of the nineteenth-century's most influential poets, today Huntington Station is an impoverished stretch of neighborhoods that are occupied by a large minority population. Crime here—particularly domestic violence—as well as drug and alcohol problems and a soaring school dropout rate—were largely endemic problems that were not seen and often not discussed outside the "Station." Bernadette has a little house there where she devotes her whole life to social service. Her own home is just about always full of foster children who are in her care. In this loving, nurturing environment, she has raised dozens of orphaned, neglected, or disadvantaged children herself. Bern's voice is a strong one in the community. As a civic activist she has spearheaded innumerable community causes through the years.

Lauren and Bernadette first met after a young boy died in a foster home in Huntington. All that was known about the child's death was that he fell off a top bunk bed, suffered a concussion, and died later in his sleep. The exact circumstances surrounding the accident were unknown. Bernadette first mentioned the situation to Brian, who passed the information along to Lauren, who, he thought, would get along well with Bernadette. But when the two women seemed to immediately bond it was more than Brian could have hoped for, especially when Lauren was diagnosed with lung cancer soon afterward. Bern was a woman of strong faith, and Lauren's relationship with her during this period was vitally important to her.

Lauren attended the child's funeral and was appalled when a fight broke out among several of the mourners. Bernadette was there to help keep the peace; she also tried to pacify a visibly shaken Lauren who thought she had seen it all. Lauren was utterly amazed by Bernadette's composure in a situation that was every bit as unpredictable as it was distressing.

Shortly after that, Bernadette organized a series of candlelight vigils to bring awareness to various issues of violence and abuse in the community. There had also recently been a rash of shootings in the neighborhood. Lauren was there to cover the vigil, but the event spawned a more in-depth story, and the paper ended up sending several other reporters to cover allegations of abuse and neglect that had been going on in various daycare facilities and children's treatment centers.

Bernadette was happy that so much was written about the problem. It generated much-needed exposure so that something would be done to start to change things for the better. As a direct result of all the articles that appeared in the paper over a period of weeks, several of those facilities were forced to shut down.

One of the stories Lauren wrote that impacted many readers, generating outrage and a call for action, was titled "Troubled Kids, Far From Home/Probing Care, Oversight at Treatment Centers." The article focused on a shy and sensitive sixteen-year-old girl, Chloe Cohen, who wrote poetry and sketched portraits and who also had "spent many of her years in special educational programs," according to Lauren's article, and was "becoming increasingly prone to emotional meltdowns." As her problems worsened, she was sent to a residential treatment center called KidsPeace. Six weeks after entering the facility, Chloe was found dead with a bathrobe belt around her neck and hanging from a metal railing on her bunk bed. Her death was ruled a suicide.

Lauren wrote, "A *Newsday* review has found that several of the institutions used by both counties have troubling records themselves: boys and girls as young as twelve have been assaulted, have committed suicide, or have been killed or molested by the workers who are charged with their care." Lauren went on to cite a number of examples of recorded cases of child abuse that had taken place at facilities that were supposed to help children deal with their problems.

"Seven months have passed since Chloe's death," Lauren's article concluded, "and Maleka Cohen (Chloe's mother) still wonders about what happened that night. More importantly, she wonders if Cohen and others like her are best served in such places."

It was around this time that Brian called Bernadette to inform her that Lauren had been diagnosed with lung cancer. He told her that Lauren wanted to see her, as a friend and a minister; Brian drove Bernadette into New York to visit Lauren at her apartment. Bernadette brought a bottle of anointing oil with her, which she gave to Lauren along with an angel figurine to watch over her, and she ministered to Lauren for most of the day.

Bernadette was a true believer in the healing properties of anointed oil, and as Lauren began her cancer treatment she would anoint herself with the oil, and she began praying more. All the while, she and Bernadette stayed in touch with each other. One thing they always talked about was the children. It was perhaps the strongest connection between them. Even when Lauren was most sick from the chemotherapy and Bernadette was ministering to her and consoling her through her own difficult time, the children remained a priority. They would discuss the welfare of certain children who were most hurting and make determinations about what they could do to help them by working in the community to create a safer, more nurturing environment for them. Bernadette knew how much their well-being meant to Lauren, and she would tell Lauren that they were going to work together again soon to help the children. It seemed to help sustain Lauren, and when her cancer went into remission, no one was happier than Bernadette.

Brian, who played such an important intermediary role in the relationship between the two women, often drove Bernadette from Long Island into the city so she could visit with and minister to Lauren. There were the occasional *Driving Miss Daisy* jokes, but Bernadette and Lauren were both indebted to Brian for bringing them together. He would take Bernadette to the hospital to visit Lauren as well as to the newsroom at *Newsday* when she was working so they could share some time together. She would often bring Lauren flowers and small gifts, and Lauren in turn would send gifts to Bernadette. Lauren became like one of Bernadette's own children, Bernadette loved her that much.

When Lauren's cancer returned and her doctors gave her no hope, Bernadette continued to minister to her. Several days before she passed away, they spent several hours together. They talked about everything, and when the subject of the end of life came up, Bernadette told Lauren that when that time came, it was in God's hands.

"That's something you have no control over," Bernadette told Lauren. "When God says it's over, then it's over. Not when the doctors say. They're not God. All we know is that right now, it's not over. We're still here together. None of us can do anything more than live for today, for the moment, really. You just keep going and you strive for tomorrow and you never give up and when God calls you home, you go to him."

In the hospital that last time, Bernadette could see that Lauren was ready. She was comfortable, not complaining, not angry or bitter. She seemed subdued, very much at peace, and if she felt any anguish or disappointment, she seemed to have come to terms with it. When Bernadette walked out of the hospital that day and left Lauren, she wondered if she would ever see her again.

As a minister, and taking into account all she had seen and been through in life, Bernadette was used to friends and loved ones passing on. Over time she had developed what she calls a "discerning" ability that told her when people were at the end of their life. She could usually recognize when that time was, but for Lauren she could not. It wasn't just Lauren's strength and determination or her will to live. Bernadette was so close to Lauren that all she saw was life when she looked at Lauren. She was going to make it because that's what Bernadette needed. She needed to be close to Lauren. She needed that relationship.

On their drive back to Huntington, Brian asked her, "Are we coming back?"

"We're coming back," Bernadette answered him, but deep in her heart she knew that would be the last time she would see Lauren alive.

Bernadette held on to everything that went on that day in the hospital and every word that was spoken between her and Lauren. Bernadette believed that God put them together for the time Lauren had left, and it was special for Lauren because she had someone she could bond with on another level.

When Lauren passed away, Bernadette thought with profound sadness, "My baby is gone." She often referred to Lauren as her baby, a love that will always be there, like a mother to a child. Bernadette recognized that the loss was not just hers, or even that of Lauren's own family and her many friends, but it was the community's loss as well. The real loss for Bernadette was that Lauren was in her life for such a short time.

When her brother contracted colon cancer, Bernadette nursed and ministered to him, and what she had learned from her relationship with Lauren, she was able to give to her brother. It was a genuine "pay it forward" moment for Bernadette. It was one thing to minister to someone when you're not hurting and going through cancer, but it's quite another when you can take what somebody else went through and tell another person, without any doubt, that they can be comfortable and at peace as well.

For Bernadette, in many ways her relationship with Lauren has not ended. She has so many memories of Lauren, and the things they said to one another come back easily. There are physical remembrances that are equally as important.

One of the gifts Lauren had given to Bernadette was an iPod. It was the first and only one she has ever owned, and to this day she has not used it. It means too much to her and is too sad a reminder of Lauren and how their time together on earth ended so soon, so she keeps it in its pristine state, just as it was the day she received it from Lauren. No so with the cancer charm bracelet that Bernadette had given Lauren, who loved it so much that Bernadette went out and got one for herself. She still wears it in Lauren's memory.

5

April Rogalski met Lauren during their sophomore year at Boston University. She moved into the Towers' International Floor where Lauren had been living. April was happy just to be out of West Campus and the large, crowded residence halls where she had spent her freshman year. Close to the sports complex, West was an ideal place to live if you were an athlete, but for April it wasn't close enough to the College of Communication.

She knew right away she would be better off at the Towers. The rooms were doubles and each floor was single-sex, with floor residents sharing a common bathroom. The elevators split the floor with four rooms in each direction. The rooms that were located in the "elevator lobby" had a little lounge area outside of them, painted a garish yellow-mustard color, with standard-issue university furniture that included a love seat, a couple of chairs, and a coffee table set directly in front of windows facing Bay State Road.

The common bathrooms were located at the intersection of the two hallways, and at the opposite ends of the floor furthest from the elevator bank there were four single-occupancy rooms facing Commonwealth Avenue. There were large windows at the end of each hallway outside the "singles."

April was in room 704 East, and she shared a wall with Lauren, who was in 706 East. Each dorm room had two small vertical windows and between them was a kind of vanity shelf with a radiator beneath it. There was a desk next to each window. The placement of the desks made it difficult to look out the window, but even if you managed to get a look outside, there wasn't much to see. All you got was a view of the West Tower. April can still accurately recall many of the details because she spent so much time there. She really enjoyed being around most of the girls on the floor, particularly Lauren, who also ended up spending a considerable amount of time in Room 704. Lauren's roommate, Mona, was a very pretty Middle Eastern girl who always had a lot of boys coming around, so when Lauren had to study or just wanted to get away, she would often go next door into April's room.

April and Lauren got along very well. They both liked to laugh and joke, sometimes just between themselves, to the point that others might think it was at their expense. They called each other by their initials, so April was AD and Lauren was LT. It was a code that only the two of them used.

What they did most was just plain talk. One of the things they sometimes talked about was having a family someday. For both girls, however, at that stage of their lives—still at school and with strong career ambitions as newswomen—having children was a distant dream, but it was something else they both shared. Children would come later, they thought, after they got out of school and conquered the world. This left them free to talk about more immediate topics, like dating and boys.

April did not have any classes with Lauren that semester. She was in the college of basic studies, taking her first two communications classes that semester. At BU, you either went right into your major or into the college of basic studies to fulfill your core requirement classes until a spot opened up in the crowded communications classes. Boston University had one of the best journalism programs in the country, so it was worth the wait. April was interested in going into broadcast journalism and had aspirations to be a television reporter.

April and Lauren were good friends over the course of their three remaining years at Boston University. Even though they did not live together after their sophomore year in the Towers, they would get together occasionally, and they shared some classes. On graduation day, the two girls found themselves together and shared a moment that left them laughing the way they had laughed so many times on the seventh floor of the Towers the first year they met.

While springtime in Boston is usually quite nice, graduation day in 1990 was drizzly, raw, and cold. Still, April and Lauren would not let it ruin their day and everything that it symbolized for them as students—leaving four years of college and experiences behind them forever as they embarked on the next step in their lives and careers. The week before their big day they had gone out together and bought beautiful dresses to wear underneath their gowns, and even though no one could see what they were wearing beneath their robes, it made them feel special, and that was all that mattered. As they walked down Emerson Field for the commencement, their heels were sinking into the mud, but they just looked at each other and laughed.

Ginny and I were on hand, of course. We were so proud of Lauren, especially since both of us had completed high school only. She had worked hard and exceled in the classroom, but she had also overcome a lot of adjustment issues early on and stuck it out. That was an invaluable part of her education, and it was a lesson that made it all worthwhile, in my opinion.

During the ceremony they sat beside each other, listening to the speakers. Suddenly something hit Lauren on the head. It struck her cap with an audible thump. April looked over and saw that it was bird droppings.

"Oh my God," April said, laughing. "A bird just shit on your head."

Lauren removed the mortarboard and looked at it in disbelief.

"That's supposed to be good luck," April said and laughed some more as Lauren banged her cap on the ground. The bird poop dropped off and she placed the mortarboard back on her head, unable to contain her own laughter as she sat there for the remainder of the graduation ceremony in the rain with a whitish-gray stain on her cap.

1990 was a year of national economic downturn, resulting in many recent college graduates finding that they were unable to obtain employment in their desired field, Lauren among them.

That summer, Lauren submitted her resume everywhere, but because of the limited amount of advertised positions available, she had few calls for interviews locally. As a result, she concluded that the potential for landing a journalism position in the current job climate was considerably greater elsewhere. Much to the dismay of her mother and me (as well as my legs and my back), she decided to move to New York City. She quickly made arrangements to stay with a friend who had previously relocated to Manhattan.

The anxiety my wife and I experienced as a result of this announcement was immense, exceeding by far the angst we had gone through during her initial days living in Boston. Our little girl moving to the Big Apple—a city noted for, among many things, all sorts of criminal activity—without a job and far from family seemed more than we would be able to handle as parents.

Despite my own reluctance, I could not stop her from doing what was probably the best thing for her career under the circumstances. I knew we had to let go. She was no longer a little girl, but a beautiful young woman capable of making her own decisions. So one weekend in late September, we loaded up a rented U-Haul van, filled it with Lauren's belongings, and off we went down I-95 south. Upon our arrival in New York, we learned that Lauren's roommate, for some unexplained reason, was moving to another location. We ended up spending the weekend cramming the van with her friend's possessions; I became an independent moving company once again.

In the days and weeks after her arrival in New York, Lauren diligently immersed herself in finding a job. Resume in hand, she "hit the ground running," visiting any and all companies that had an entry-level journalism position available.

Though Lauren and April went their separate ways, they stayed in close contact over the next few years. April visited Lauren in New York when she was attending Columbia, and they were bridesmaids at each other's weddings. April recalls clearly the old Irish blessing that Lauren recited during her wedding reception. "May the happiest day of your past," Lauren said, raising her glass, "be the saddest day of your future."

Soon they began to slowly drift apart, as often happens with college friends. April started graduate school to get her MBA and started a family at the same time. The years went by. When she found out that Lauren had died, she was deeply saddened by the news. She remembered the conversations they had had in college about children and how Lauren had wanted to have a family of her own. In learning that Lauren had not experienced the delight and wonder of being a mother, April began to cry.

Six

Small Gestures Can
Be a Huge Booster

For many people with cancer, validation of the difficult time is all they want. Some call it emotional triage. One woman friend who went through a six-year battle with cancer said she never wanted a pity party, but she was comforted when friends would acknowledge how lousy and unfair things were at times. She said she was sick of the chirpy people who treated her cancer as if it were nothing more than a broken ankle.

Hope said friends and family should validate that it is normal to feel depressed at times and that cancer patients

*shouldn't feel inadequate or guilty for not having a more
positive attitude. And yes, acknowledge that it is OK to be
terrified. If I wasn't scared, one of my doctors once told me
as I once sobbed in his office, he would have ordered a psy-
chiatric evaluation.*

*Perhaps more than anything, showing up for the person
means the most to those who are sick. There have been people I never expected to show up, who did. And, of course, my
friends, family and co-workers who have more than stuck
around. My friend Monica was always willing to accompany me to a doctor's appointment. She would often show up
with prepared food so I wouldn't have to cook.*

*My friends Tomoeh and Archie always seem to get it
right. It's not what they say, but it's often what they do.
When I was stuck in intensive care at a Boston hospital after a life-threatening infection from chemo gone awry, the
couple shuffled 40 blocks uptown to my apartment in New
York to pick up the mail and check on things. In anticipation
of my arrival home a month later, without being asked, they
arrived the day before and cleaned the place top to bottom.*

—From *Newsday*, "Life, with Cancer," December 19, 2006,
"Small Gestures Can Be a Huge Booster," by Lauren Terrazzano

1

Lauren had been with *Newsday* several years before Dawn
Mackeen joined the staff. She was familiar with Lauren's writing,

of course, and she was well aware of the respect everyone in the newsroom had for her. As a successful female journalist who was still young and had won a number of awards, including a Pulitzer, Lauren was someone Dawn looked up to as a role model.

Dawn sat close to Lauren in the newsroom, and they would talk occasionally about nonwork-related topics. While Dawn covered a wide range of health care and aging issues, including anything at all that had to do with hospitals and senior citizens, there was some overlap with the social services stories Lauren wrote, but she never thought they would have the opportunity to actually work together until, quite unexpectedly, they did.

Adults with disabilities who were being mistreated was an area where they had some common ground, and in the fall of 2003 when Dawn began an investigation into how poorly some Suffolk County assisted-living facilities were being run, she happened to mention the story she was working on to Lauren. She told Lauren a little bit about the assignment and some of the problems she had uncovered, including some suspected neglect and abuse concerns. That was enough for Lauren, and when Dawn explained how she was still in the early stages of the project, still discovering new cases and corruption the deeper she probed, Lauren become visibly excited. Dawn could practically hear Lauren's journalistic wheels turning as Lauren peppered her with questions which, for the most part, Dawn could not answer.

Lauren asked Dawn if she could join her in the investigation, and even though it was in the form of a question, it was really more of a statement, a pronouncement of fact. As far as Dawn was concerned, it was already a done deal. She welcomed the opportunity to work alongside Lauren.

"This is really serious," Lauren told her, recognizing the potential for a much bigger story. "Let's do this. Let's do this really big. I'll work with you and we can turn it into a series."

Lauren's excitement continued to grow as she suggested they immediately talk to the editors, who approved the project practically on the spot. Lauren could not wait to get started and neither could Dawn, who was fired up by Lauren's enthusiasm. The two began to discuss the different ways they might approach the story, the angles they could take, the sources they could employ.

Dawn recognized that the adrenalin rush that drove Lauren and stoked her passion was not something that arose from a desire for personal achievement or recognition; Lauren really believed that an in-depth investigative story would do a lot of good, help a lot of families who would remove their loved ones from these facilities, and perhaps shut some of them down so that no one else would suffer the same abuses and indignities.

Dawn and Lauren ended up in the investigative unit together and began work on the story. They lived close to each other on the Upper West Side and drove to work together every day. The commute to the Long Island office was long and arduous, taking anywhere from forty minutes, sometimes a lot more, depending on the traffic. It provided a great opportunity for the two journalists to get to know each other. They would take turns driving, though Lauren would always get most of what Dawn called the "Massachusetts days," referring to those days when it was snowing. Dawn was from California, so she would leave the driving when winter weather was in the fore-cast to Lauren, who had no fear of navigating the already congested city streets that became even more constricted and hazardous when snow would begin to accumulate. With coffees in hand, they had plenty of time to talk about the story, but also about other things that women talk about, such as dating.

As their investigative work got into full swing, they practically lived together. They holed up in the investigative unit office and worked long hours starting early in the morning and finishing late most nights for the eight months they worked on the story. "Hey, babe," was a typical greeting Dawn would hear from Lauren when one of them walked into a room where the other one was working.

Lauren's instincts were quickly proved right. It was a major story that affected the lives of many people, almost too many to keep track of. But Lauren didn't want any of the team to lose sight of the individuals involved—the flesh and blood people behind what they were doing—so she devised a simple but effective way for them to keep everything in perspective. In the investigative office, she set up a large cork bulletin board where the team would post the photographs of each victim of abuse that they uncovered in the various assisted-living facilities they looked into. The photographs put a human face on the suffering that was taking place, often unbeknownst to the families of the victims.

Lauren worked her sources and found families that had filed civil suits or criminal complaints against assisted-living facilities. She spoke with the victims themselves or their loved ones. She interviewed people in the health department. The team's probing focused on how residents who were suffering from dementia were being treated, or in some cases mistreated, in these facilities. Eden pursued her police contacts for cases of reported violence against elderly residents in assisted-living facilities and combed through missing-persons reports of anyone with dementia that had been filed with the police. Some residents were shown to have been physically mistreated by assisted-living staff members, a few even violently attacked, either by other patients or members of the staff.

Dawn focused her efforts primarily on issues involving health and medicine. Everyone residing in an assisted-living setting had some physical disability or a diminished or impaired mental process, sometimes both. Their very lives depended on a personal regimen of care that usually included prescribed medications that needed to be taken according to precise specifications. These basic needs, it was discovered, were often not being met; the investigation found some residents missed doses of their medication for long periods of time.

As more cases of neglect and abuse against elderly people residing in assisted-living facilities were uncovered, Lauren made sure each of them was represented with a photograph on the corkboard in the investigative unit. If no current picture of an individual could be found, Lauren would get her camera out and take a snapshot of the person herself. With each additional photograph, the work they were all doing on the story seemed to become that much more important. At least it did for Dawn. That was probably what Lauren had intended when she bought the corkboard and put it up in the investigations room. Over time, the images of the elderly victims covered it so completely that some photographs had to be taped to the frame and the wall around the board.

Dawn left *Newsday* in 2004, shortly after the paper ran the assisted-living series and around the time Lauren got sick, and then left New York altogether in 2006, heading back home to California. She saw Lauren shortly before she passed away. Although Lauren was having trouble breathing, was bedridden, and had a distended abdomen, she was still so full of life it was hard for Dawn to believe that anything could keep her down for long, let alone stop her. Dawn told Lauren about a book she was writing and Lauren became very excited. It was almost the same excitement Dawn remembered Lauren having for the assisted-living series when she first proposed the idea. Lauren wanted to know who Dawn's agent and editor were and all the details about Dawn's book. Lauren said that she had always wanted to write a book of her own one day.

2

Before she became a friend and colleague of Lauren's at *Newsday*, Amanda Harris knew just about all there was to know about Lauren, who at the time was still at graduate student. Lauren had applied for the Anne O'Hare McCormick Memorial Scholarship, which had been established by several members of the Newswomen's Club of New York to honor *New York Times* journalist Anne O'Hare McCormick following her death in 1954. O'Hare McCormick had gained prominence while reporting from Europe in the 1930s. She chronicled Adolf Hitler's rise to power and interviewed many of the power brokers and leaders of that era. In 1937 she became the first woman to win a Pulitzer prize for foreign correspondence. She served as a vice president of the Newswomen's Club of New York for several years and was the first woman to serve on the *New York Times* editorial board.

The purpose of the fund is to give scholarships to outstanding women students at Columbia University's Graduate School of Journalism. In 1994 Lauren won the award, and Amanda recalls being very impressed with Lauren's application. Besides Lauren's biography and list of references, the application contained a writing sample in which she explained why she wanted to become a journalist and what she hoped to achieve. Her words articulated not only her ambition but a keen understanding of some of the professional obstacles she would face, particularly as a woman in the field; these were considerations that most journalism students rarely think about as they embark on their careers.

Amanda had grown up in Manhattan and had also graduated from Columbia's journalism school prior to being hired by *Newsday*. She started out as a reporter at the paper's Long Island desk. She later served as a correspondent in Albany before becoming a business reporter, then a business editor, then state editor responsible for all state government-related news. In 1985 she became an editor for the city edition of *Newsday* before going back to Melville, New York, ten years later to join the paper's elite investigative team in Long Island. That's where she was in 2003 when she first heard about the assisted-living story. The investigative unit office was abuzz with the news that Lauren and Dawn were teaming up to look into an interesting and tragic story involving the questionable care provided to elderly residents of assisted-living facilities.

What Amanda found interesting was that in recent years there had been an increasing number of housing developments popping up all around Long Island that had gone into the "assisted-living business." Perhaps taking advantage of a graying American population, these facilities fell into a gray area, legally, because they were neither apartments nor licensed nursing homes but something in between. In a lot of cases, the cost to live in one of them was as much as some nursing homes, though they provided none of the care that many elderly people living alone need to sustain themselves. The trouble was that there were numerous incidents involving residents with dementia walking out of the residences unnoticed and wandering around outside, putting themselves and others at risk, some even dying as a consequence. The number of elderly people living in such facilities was staggering. There were hundreds of thousands of them, and the figure was increasing. The preliminary findings were turning up a lot of evidence of abuse, more than enough to support a full investigation.

Lauren would temporarily relocate to the investigative office from the early stages of story's development through its completion. The large central room was quiet and removed from the noise and bustle of the newsroom.

For nearly a year, Amanda witnessed Lauren's personal outrage and compassion for all the people affected by what was revealed during the course of the assisted-living abuse investigation. From the moment she took Dawn's story to her editors for approval as an in-depth investigative series to the date of publication of the final story in the series, her drive never faltered.

While Lauren went out into the field to conduct interviews, Amanda did a lot of the research into the records of the various facilities and filed various Freedom of Information requests, including all the FCC filings.

Though Amanda may have had the most experience of anyone on the team, she realized that this story would not be hers to lead and she was fine with that. She was happy to assist and provide whatever research information she could. It was a big story. Egos and byline credits aside, all that mattered was completing the research and having a viable story in the end. Amanda had been with *Newsday* for thirty years, and although she did not know exactly when she would be moving on from the paper, it could be anytime. This was the kind of story she would have been proud to go out with.

Shortly after *Newsday* ran the assisted-living series, Amanda had taken a buyout and left the paper. She later told me that her work with Lauren ended up being one of the more personally rewarding stories she ever worked on.

3

Individuals with dementia, and their treatment, became a major focus of the series. The first installment, which Lauren wrote, was called "The Wanderers." It included detailed reports of residents who had wandered out of facilities without even being noticed until they were discovered, lost and disoriented, often barefoot and half-naked, sometimes miles away from the facilities, at train stations, on the Long Island Expressway, some even in Manhattan. There were a number of people who were seriously injured, including as many as seven who died as a result of this "wandering," which was happening with regularity in communities where assisted-living facilities were located.

Lauren interviewed the family of one elderly woman who had walked unnoticed out of a center on a cold December night and stumbled and fell into a fish pond on the property not far from the front entrance. Aides eventually noticed her in the icy water and pulled her out, alive but suffering from severe hypothermia. She developed a lung infection that killed her a couple of weeks later.

Lack of proper care caused the death of other residents. One documented case involved a seventy-five-year-old woman with dementia who died of heart disease after missing nineteen doses of her prescribed medication.

There were other cases of personal property being reported missing. One ninety-seven-year-old great-grandmother had a diamond engagement ring that she wore every day before it suddenly disappeared.

The overall problem was due in large part to a patchwork of outdated regulations in the state of New York pertaining to the assisted-living industry. As advances in medicine and health care were allowing people to live longer and with greater independence, assisted-living facilities were popping up everywhere. Safety and security were already major issues in the industry. Lauren found in her research that as much as 50 percent of the population of assisted-living centers nationally had dementia, including 3,500 on Long Island alone. With so many of the residents suffering from various forms of dementia, things would only get worse.

The fact that these facilities were not equipped to handle residents with dementia and other serious health conditions that require special supervision and medical care is not surprising. At this time, governmental health and safety regulations played little or no role in how these facilities were run because they were classified as "adult care" facilities. Because of this designation, they were legally permitted to operate under guidelines that were meant to pertain to a younger group of people under rules that had been written more than thirty years earlier. In the 1970s, the Department of Social Services (DSS) was the governing body responsible for instituting state legislation, not the health department, so mandates such as the requirement to have a nurse on the premises at all times does not apply to these facilities. In a few instances, Lauren and the investigative team found that some facilities were not licensed at all.

Because these centers were free and clear of health department guidelines and regulation enforcement, the assisted-living industry on Long Island and across the entire state of New York was getting away with murder, sometimes literally. The inadequate treatment and lack of proper care only perpetuated further neglect and abuse. Many family members did not know the full extent of the problems in these centers and felt great guilt; in many cases, the children of the elderly simply could not care for their parents or aging relatives at home but thought they were putting them in a safe environment. That was not always the case.

The person who provided most of the research for the *Newsday* stories, and without whose work the series might never have been possible, was Eden Laikin. She worked hard and was good at every-thing she did. Through the years, the paper gave her more and more responsibility, but she lacked the confidence to fulfill her dream of becoming a full-fledged journalist, at least until Lauren came along and joined *Newsday*.

The two women met at a work conference but did not become chummy right away. Much later, Eden would ask Lauren why they hadn't become friends sooner and Lauren admitted that she thought Eden did not like her, which scared her off. Eden was surprised, because she had been intimidated by Lauren, who was a real journal-ist, and Eden didn't think they had anything in common. They came to discover that they had quite a few similarities.

As they got closer, they realized how much they both wanted to work on the investigative side of reporting. Often, as Lauren began developing a story, she would come to Eden for research help (which was what Eden was doing a great deal of at the time, anyway) and they would talk about the kinds of investigative stories they would like to pursue. Eden was frustrated because she was no closer now to being an investigative journalist than she had been when she was making copies in her first days at *Newsday*. And although she was working in the investigative unit when she joined Lauren and Dawn on the assisted-living report, she still had not done any significant contributive writing of her own. She would go out and do the report-ing, and then pass the information on for someone else to write. That all changed when she began to work closely with Lauren on the assisted-living story.

Eden owes a lot to Lauren for her development into the journalist that she eventually became. Lauren constantly encouraged her to write her own pieces. So convinced was Lauren that Eden could be an investigative journalist that Eden began to believe it herself. When she ending up writing her first solo story, Lauren called her from home to tell her how proud she was of her—the kind of thing that a parent might say to a child. Lauren helped her immensely with her first dozen stories and was right by her side whenever she needed Lauren for advice or just to listen. She helped Eden not only by giving her pointers on interviewing and on writing techniques but also on how to deal with editors.

Eden feels she learned most about how to be a good journalist while she was working alongside Lauren on the assisted-living series. Eden observed that it was never enough for Lauren just to speak on the phone with the people or the families that she wrote about in her stories. She needed to get together with them in person, face to face. Eden took note of how Lauren spent her time on the phone, particularly with family members of those who had died; these were not merely social calls just to see how they were doing. And sometimes the families would call Lauren, the conversations lasting more than an hour on occasion. Eden observed Lauren quietly address these grieving people by first name and speak with them like she had known them for years.

Lauren possessed an enormous amount of genuine empathy and compassion. The tears she shed with people were real. Witnessing it firsthand, Eden understood that this was what allowed her to connect so deeply with victims' families during the most difficult of times. Lauren took great pains to use just the right words to describe their tragedies. And this all came out in her writing for anyone to read and feel the same emotions she experienced in reporting the story.

At one point during the course of the assisted-living investigation, Eden and Lauren went together to one of the centers to see for themselves what it was like there and how the residents lived. They ended up meeting and talking with a kind old gentleman who seemed starved for attention and personal interaction. Lauren engaged him in conversation for quite a while, and on at least one further occasion that Eden knew about, Lauren went back to the center to play checkers with him. His photo wound up on the top of the corkboard in the investigative office; looking up and seeing him there always put a smile on Lauren's face. It was one of the few fond memories Eden had of her visits to any of the centers they visited. Most of what she saw inside their walls was not easy to look at: frail, infirm people, many with dementia, who looked frightened and lost or seemed sad and helpless. It was difficult for Lauren as well, who had seen much more than Eden had. It affected them so much that during a visit to one particular center they simply had to leave.

Eden and Lauren spent a lot of time together during those months and became even closer as a result. Eden lived on Long Island, and on days when they put in extra hours, Lauren would frequently stay overnight at Eden's house. Eden noticed how Lauren's expression changed the instant they started heading away from the city. "This is where I'd like to live," Lauren would say as they drove farther east. Even though she was a city girl now, Lauren loved staying at Eden's house. She would wake up early in the morning with a big smile on her face as she looked out the window at the grass and the trees. But that ended, too, and things went back to the way they were.

When their investigative work was done, their lives went back to normal, but much anticipation remained. *Newsday* editors were hopeful that the investment of time and resources would pay off, but no one on the investigative team was worried. They all knew that what they had was powerful and informative, as well as shocking and tragic.

By examining the full scope of dangers that existed for elderly patients in assisted-living centers on Long Island, the eight-month investigation that resulted in a four-part series in *Newsday* was successful in what it had hoped to achieve all along as well as a realization of the vision Lauren had when Dawn first told her about the elderly abuse she had uncovered. The investigation had a major impact not only on Long Island readers and among people whose loved ones were living in these facilities, but it also caught the attention of lawmakers in Albany.

Because of the revelations of appalling mistreatment and criminal conduct, and the attention that the story garnered around New York, sweeping changes were made in the way assisted-living facilities were licensed and evaluated. Within a couple months of the series' appearance in *Newsday*, legislation was drafted to toughen state inspections of these facilities. Later that same year, New York Governor George Pataki signed into law the Assisted Living Reform Act. This comprehensive and historic assisted-living reform legislation provided New York senior citizens with greater protections and improved long-term care options.

In the past, Lauren had written stories that motivated individuals or organizations into taking action, but this was the first time that a story she worked on resulted directly in changes being instituted by government agencies. That Lauren helped make it safer for dementia patients living in facilities all across the state was something of which she was very proud.

Lauren had learned about her illness around the same time that the team's work was recognized for all its achievements, but she never let that stop her from sharing the joy of what they had accomplished together. There was one particular award dinner that was memorable above all others, but it wasn't the trophy or the parchment with their names in fancy calligraphy that made it stand out. Eden, Lauren, and Dawn found themselves traveling together by train across town to the award dinner that night, and they had the best time on the trip. They laughed a lot, they cried, and they talked about all kinds of things. They put aside Lauren's grim cancer diagnosis for those several hours on the train and just laughed and had "girl talk," as if they didn't have a care in the world.

For Eden, the train ride was much like life itself; it was the journey that mattered most, not the destination.

4

Graziela Terrazzano was Lauren's paternal grandmother. Everyone called her Gracie, but Lauren called her Nona Grace. She was born and lived her entire life in a three-family walk-up in one of Boston's first Italian neighborhoods. Lubec Street, on the corner of Porter Street, was less than a mile from Logan Airport. The Mass Pike, I-90, was practically in the backyard. Despite all this activity around the house, Nona Grace was a woman who seldom strayed too far from those East Boston streets or left the confines of the comfortable home where she had raised two boys. The one and only time Nona Grace left Boston and the country was a trip she made to Italy in 1975. Her three sisters, Lauren's great-aunts Rosie, Fannie, and Emma, lived below her on the second floor in the front and rear apartments. The first floor had belonged to Nona Grace's parents before they passed.

Lauren spent many happy times at 62 Lubec Street with her grandmother and cousins. Nona Grace had potted tomato plants on the tarred flat roof of the house, and when she tended them Lauren and her cousins loved going up with her. They called it "tar beach." In the summertime heat, the air was thick with the cloying aroma of ripe tomatoes and the searing smell of hot tar. The homegrown tomatoes were used to make Nona Grace's pasta sauce, or "gravy," as most Italian Americans called it.

From the rooftop the sound of the planes coming and going overhead was so loud it shook the tomatoes on the vines. Lauren used to look up at the planes and think about all the exciting and wonderful places they were going. As a little girl she would imagine that she was on board, traveling to some exotic land to write a story for a major newspaper or magazine.

Going to her grandmother's house was an adventure for Lauren when she was young. She would spend some of her summer vacation days there. Her grandmother would take her downtown for a visit to the Boston Public Gardens or the famed Boston Common, the Hub's equivalent of New York's Central Park, where they would always have a traditional ride on the swan boats at the duck pond.

Some nights Lauren would stay over in Nona Grace's three-room flat. It was small and cramped, but Lauren didn't mind a bit. The bathroom wasn't even in the apartment, it was down the hall. What might have been an inconvenience for some people was for Lauren all part of the allure and mystery of being away from home. For her, it was like visiting another country. It was where she developed a love of foreign language, as Italian was spoken most often in the house. Her grandmother spoke English. Her grandfather, Francesco, spoke with his own unique dialect, a mixture of English and Italian that was harder to understand than either language alone. He used to call her "Laurenna" in his broken-English accent.

Unlike Nona Grace, Francesco Terrazzano was quiet and reserved, but he loved Lauren more than anything. He could never do enough for her; she was the only female grandchild in the family. He spent a lot of his time around the stove and was a very good cook himself. He would cook to order any special dish that Lauren wanted. If he wasn't in the kitchen, Lauren would be sure to find him in his green leather armchair in the living room reading the paper or watching television. This was also where Lauren would sit and read her Nancy Drew books.

While her grandfather's dishes were always a treat, Nona Grace's cooking represented something more. For Lauren, she was the link between family generations, and so much of what she communi- cated was through her cooking. She had a no-nonsense way about everything she did. She wore a sleeveless housedress most days, even in the dead of winter, with sensible leather shoes and her signature apron. When someone had a problem, food was her antidote for all the troubles of life.

"Hungry?" Nona Grace would ask as soon as Lauren walked in the door. But Lauren never had time to answer before food appeared on the kitchen table as if by magic. At a moment's notice, Nona Grace would lay out a veritable banquet that might include a tossed salad smothered with fresh cucumber and tomato slices, homemade minestrone, pasta with meatballs and *bresaola*, either her meat lasagna or eggplant parmigiani, and of course her famous *pizzelles* for dessert.

They would sit at the kitchen table, which was always covered with a clear plastic tablecloth so as to keep food stains from the faux-wooden tabletop. After a meal they would sit and eat *pizzelles* for dessert. The thin, wafflelike cookies were lovingly made with an old-fashioned iron. Covered with a light coating of powdered sugar, though sometimes glazed with honey or decorated with colored sprinkles, these treats are a perennial Italian tradition. Nona Grace's recipe had been passed down from her mother and her mother's mother. This simple, crispy cookie, indented with its classic stencil-like pattern, sometimes with snowflake or spider web designs, sustained her and her family through poverty and the hardships of the Great Depression.

Though the recipe seemed simple enough, with a batter consisting of eggs, flour, milk, a hint of vanilla and just a twist of anise, the process was somewhat involved. The heavy, antique iron had to be heated on the stovetop for about fifteen minutes before batter was dropped over the scorching wrought iron template. Because they could only be made one at a time, it took just about a full afternoon to make a plateful. The tricky part came when the batter cooked and the wafer cookie reached a perfect golden brown. With a spatula, the *pizzelle* had to be carefully pried off the hot iron or else it would break into a million pieces on the counter. With just a flick of the wrist, Nona Grace's *pizzelles* would drop off the iron perfectly before being placed on a baker's rack for cooling.

When Lauren was a student at Boston University, Nona Grace was sick and battling breast cancer. Lauren would take the T (Boston's transit system) into East Boston to help her clean and straighten up her apartment. With limited mobility in her arms, and weakened by surgery and chemotherapy, Grace was unable to do the things she used to, such as vacuuming and getting dressed. But every time Lauren came over, there would be a plate of *pizzelles* waiting for her. Comfort and warmth on a chipped, flowered plate. Lauren never knew how she managed to pull that off. They would end up sitting around the kitchen table with fresh *pizzelles* and a cup of tea or coffee. Lauren didn't know what to say or do. Her grandmother was the one who always made things right, and she usually did so without saying a word. During this time, while Lauren was at school, consumed with the trials and tribulations of young adulthood, Nona Grace would send care packages of food that included, of course, her *pizzelles*, to Lauren's dorm.

Years later, when Lauren was diagnosed with cancer herself, she wished that she could be transported back in time to sit once again at the familiar kitchen table at Nona Grace's house. She would have liked nothing more than to be given another opportunity to talk to her grandmother about her illness so she wouldn't have to suffer through it so silently in the last years of her life.

Just one last time, to have a plate of *pizzelles* between them, Lauren was sure that everything would have been okay, at least for that moment.

Seven

Feeling on Top of Everything, Briefly

I needed to feel alive. There's nothing like climbing a mountain to do that. Even if it's only a 4-mile climb that wends its way through the famed Appalachian Trail.

In the old days it would take me 90 minutes to get to the peak, which rewards hikers with an observation tower and magnificent views of the Bear Mountain Bridge and the Hudson River. Bear Mountain, incidentally, has few bears. It is named because the mountain is said to resemble a sleeping one.

"There must be a column in this somewhere," my friend

Monica suggested as we clambered along the icy trail, holding onto trees and hiking sticks so we wouldn't butt-slide down the steep mountain path.

As we climbed I remembered getting up there once, picnic lunch in hand, and seeing the tops of the Twin Towers off in the distance. That was just a few days before Sept. 11, 2001.

In 2005, 10 months after my first surgery, to remove the lung, I somehow managed to get 40 wonderful reporter friends (not a small feat, since we aren't the most athletic bunch) and their families to climb the mountain as a fundraiser for underinsured lung cancer patients. We celebrated at the summit with catered sandwiches and chocolate cookies.

The climb on this March day was a little different. It was icy on most of the trail, and nippy in the areas shaded by the tall evergreens. Whenever I got tired, my husband would grab my arm and pull me up the path. Monica offered plentiful words of encouragement while carrying my pack, all the while threatening to kill me for putting myself in such a precarious situation.

In a sweep of melodrama, I sat on a dry log and told them to go on without me. Perhaps the illness simply has taken its toll. But more than two hours later, we did, in fact, make it to the top. The icy, cold top. Victory. There was no one else up there.

A few days later, my white blood cells plummeted, an occasional side effect of cancer treatment. Perhaps the exertion *of the hike didn't help. I was contemplating not writing a column this week.*

But as I write this, I am bored, sitting in a hospital bed listening to the rhythmic sound of an IV pump as it transports fluids and antibiotics through my veins. Silly me.

That's the thing about cancer. There are a lot of peaks and valleys. One minute you're on the top of the mountain, the next minute you're at the base of the trail again.

—From *Newsday*, "Life, with Cancer," March 20, 2007,
"Feeling on Top of Everything, Briefly," by Lauren Terrazzano

1

In September 2005 Lauren visited her longtime friend Dina in Guatemala. After a year in which Lauren had gone through a rigorous regimen of chemotherapy and radiation as well as major surgery to remove a lung, she planned the trip to Central America to relax and have fun. As usual with Lauren, there was always a story angle. Lauren would constantly ask Dina questions about the current state of affairs in her country. The two of them talked about these things a lot because they were of interest to both of them. They shared their ideas and thoughts about journalism, particularly the differences between journalism in the United States and Guatemala, where members of the press had to work under very difficult conditions and had to continuously defend their right to freedom of expression. Such rights, as well as the right of the Guatemalan people to information and to denounce violations of their rights, were not guaranteed.

Sometimes Lauren would find a story, as she did six years earlier when she visited Dina around the same time that the Guatemala
Truth Commission report was released. Other times a story would
find Lauren. This time it was a little of both, only it was not the political climate of the nation that would become the feature.

Several months earlier, Lauren had gone to the Bahamas along
with several of her closest friends—Leah, Tomoeh, Monica, and Sylvia—whom she referred to as her "caseworkers." While she was still
in treatment, she promised her friends, who had been by her side
the whole time, that once she recovered and was well enough she
was going to take all of them to the Bahamas as a show of gratitude.
True to her word, in June when she was feeling strong and healthy
again, they enjoyed a four-night vacation on Paradise Island, visiting
the Atlantis Resort and staying at the Beach Club. They had dinner
on the beach, Lauren rode the dolphins, they celebrated Tomoeh's
thirtieth birthday, and the girls just had one big party. It was a special
week that none of them will ever forget.

That year, the Atlantic hurricane season had been one of the most
active on record. Hurricane Katrina had hit the U.S. Gulf Coast only
a month before, devastating New Orleans as well as other parts of
Louisiana, Mississippi, and Alabama.

By the time Lauren arrived in Guatemala, the Caribbean had
already given birth to Tropical Depression 20, which was slowly
evolving into Hurricane Stan, the eleventh hurricane of the season.
As the category two storm bore down on southern Mexico and Central America in early October, Lauren found herself in the path of
destruction. Downgraded to tropical storm status once it slammed

into the Mexican state of Veracruz on October 4, the system had plenty of destructive power remaining. The real punch for most inland areas came in the form of precipitation. Stan was embedded in a larger nontropical system of rainstorms that dropped torrential rain in its wake.

The October 1 eruption of the Santa Ana volcano, located about 150 miles away in El Salvador, compounded the problem, contributing to more destructive flooding and subsequent mudslides than all the rain from the storm. The large volume of water fell on the mountainous regions of the country and loosened a mixture of saturated volcanic ash and subsoil on the downward slopes, triggering deadly landslides that jeopardized the lives of anyone living in the villages below.

The Mayan township of Panabaj, located on the edge of Lake Atitlan in the western highlands of Guatemala, lay in the direct path of a massive mudflow half a mile wide and fifteen to twenty feet high. The wall of mud and debris came thundering down the hillsides and buried everything in a tomb of wet dirt, rocks, and uprooted trees.

Lauren was at a safe enough distance inland, but when she learned of the human tragedy unfolding in another part of the country, she felt she had to do something. There were people who needed help and had suffered tremendous losses. Lauren wanted to know that the flood victims were getting the help they needed and that their stories did not go untold. There was no way she was not going to the impoverished Guatemalan provinces that were most affected by the mudslides, and all Dina could do was help her with her own connections.

Lauren was on the phone, calling everyone on Dina's source list until she managed to convince the U.S. Army Southern Command to allow her to accompany them on a mission of mercy. While Dina stayed behind, Lauren flew on missions totaling more than fifteen hours aboard a Chinook helicopter alongside four young American soldiers. She helped them deliver relief aid, including food and water and medical supplies, to the many displaced residents of the devastated mountain villages. Situated at elevations of more than a mile above sea level, many of the villages could only be reached by military helicopter.

Dina was amazed that Lauren would be so determined to work, given everything she had been through over the last twelve months.

"I don't think I would have given up a day of my vacation if the world was coming to an end," Dina later joked with Lauren.

Dina saw how Lauren had become increasingly conscious about time as a cancer survivor. She didn't want to waste a single moment. There were a lot of things she wanted to do, many goals she had left to accomplish. She had always jumped at any opportunity to make a bigger mark in her career, but this was different. She had never reported from abroad previously, and she knew that this would be a real opportunity for her to show the editors at *Newsday* that she could handle anything. Working as a foreign correspondent was something Lauren had been thinking about a lot since returning to work, and she had been lobbying her editors to get her an assignment. She was eager to show the people at the international desk just what she was capable of doing if given the chance. Dina didn't think anybody doubted Lauren's abilities, but her bosses thought that it would be best for her to remain close to home until she was at full strength and could better handle the rigors of travel associated with foreign correspondence work. Dina knew that this was what Lauren had been told by *Newsday*, and that she was not at all happy with their decision. Lauren thought this story would give them something more to think about.

Lauren and the U.S. Army Southern Command arrived at a scene of complete and utter devastation. Large boulders and a forest full of trees encased in mud had roared down the slope like a freight train and destroyed everything in its path. Hundreds of villagers were instantly killed, many of them children. This heartbreaking fact, more than anything else, compelled Lauren to find out everything she could and to help make sure everyone was taken care of.

Hurricane Stan was responsible for more than 2,100 deaths in four Central American countries: Mexico, El Salvador, Guatemala, and Nicaragua. In Panabaj alone, a Guatemalan Indian community on the outskirts of Santiago Atitlán in Sololá that was buried under a massive mudflow, the dead and missing (and presumed dead) surpassed one thousand. However, when government troops tried to enter the community to help dig out victims, the residents turned them away. With the 1990 state-sponsored massacre of thirteen villagers still fresh in their minds, the townspeople refused their help in the recovery effort and conducted the search on their own. There has always been a very strong resistance among the members of this Indian society to any interference in their culture. All the mudslide victims were Sutujil Indians. There were only about 100,000 Sutujil Indians in the country, and all of them lived in communities on the shores of Lake Atitlan. This disaster was a severe blow to these people, but they wanted to tend to their own. The hundreds of Mayan villagers, however, using an assortment of basic handheld tools, including shovels, picks, and axes to unearth victims, were overwhelmed by the task. They were forced to give up their efforts completely when experts advised them to suspend their digging because of the ever-present danger that the unstable earth would collapse again.

Community leaders asked that the area be declared a cemetery. In essence, they were attempting to disinter mudslide victims for immediate burial. "Panabaj will no longer exist," Panabaj mayor Diego Esquina was quoted in the story Lauren wrote. "We are tired. We no longer know where to dig. The bodies are so rotted that they can no longer be identified. They will only bring disease."

Guatemalan vice president Eduardo Stein promised that steps were being taken, as a sanitary measure, to give towns the legal authority to declare the buried areas cemeteries. In addition, the government asked the United Nations for a multimillion-dollar aid package because its own emergency response funds were insufficient to cover the cost of the crisis.

2

The loss of life in Guatemala to the storm and mudslides was catastrophic by any measure, but once more Lauren's focus became the children of the overrun villages. Many children were orphaned when both parents were lost in the mudslides. At least twenty-three children were orphaned in the village of Panabaj.

At that time, Dina could see that Lauren was constantly torn between the things she wanted to do and the things she had to do; sometimes there were conflicts. This was just the latest example.

Lauren's reporting on Hurricane Stan's impact on Guatemala, including the subsequent mudslide devastation, would have provided *Newsday* with at least a week's worth of stories to compete with anything the other New York papers had. The entombed Guatemalan villages, the dramatic helicopter ride with American soldiers—these were headline-grabbers, front-page material. Lauren knew that her editors would have been thrilled with any story she filed on the storm, but she wanted to focus on the Panabaj orphans and the story that developed from her reporting on the child welfare crisis in that country. In the end, that was what she did.

This was a passionate and personal subject for Lauren. She was close to several people who had an adopted child, including Sylvia Adcock, and Lauren got to see close up just how cherished an experience it was for the adoptive parents. Adopting a child was a secret desire she confided to only a few close friends, including Dina. She was single at this time, and fighting a life-threatening illness, so it was not something she would have been considering in any real way. Still, the thought persisted.

Dina had mentioned to Lauren that she was friends with a nun, Madre Inés Ayau, who ran a local orphanage. She told Lauren that Madre Ayau would often help foreigners adopt Guatemalan children, always in a safe and legal way. This was important because even then there was very little regulation of international adoptions in Guatemala, and there had been reports coming out for years about disreputable organizations involved in child trafficking and "children farms."

Of course, Lauren would not have had anything to do with organizations that victimized children in any way, but Madre Ayau was a safe and reliable option. She did, however, have several inflexible conditions of her own, the first being that adoptive parents had to be married, which effectively eliminated Lauren from consideration. But Madre Ayau did become a major source for her story, which appeared in *Newsday* on October 22, 2005.

Lauren sat down with the children. She wanted to get to know them, even though they didn't speak the same language. Even for Lauren, who could comprehend a number of foreign languages, communication was a problem, as many of the children were of Mayan descent and spoke their native language rather than Spanish. But Lauren mostly shared smiles and food with them. She absolutely fell in love with a little girl with glasses named Anabela, who was five years old. Anabela and her eight-year-old brother, Vicente, were in their home with their mother and father when they heard the rumbling start. It got louder and louder very quickly, and before they knew it, everything just went black. Their parents were swept away and killed, while the children somehow managed to survive. Anabela and Vicente were staying with other family members who were not expected to be able to keep them because they themselves were so poor.

Other children who were orphaned by the storm were in the same predicament. If no one came forward for them, they were freed for adoption and would probably wind up in either a new wave of government-run children's "protection" shelters or in established, church-run orphanages, several of which are located in Guatemala City. One of these was the Hogar Rafael Ayau, among the city's oldest orphanages and home to nearly a hundred children. This was where Madre Inés Ayau, a Christian Orthodox nun, awaited the children of the disaster.

The walled, ochre-colored orphanage rises up out of one of the city's worst neighborhoods, adjacent to a shop that sells toilet fixtures and amid prostitutes who hang out on the corner of a crowded street filled with old public buses spewing caustic black smoke into the air. But just inside the walls of the orphanage is an oasis of green space, dormitories, and a chapel.

Madre Ayau told Lauren that empty cribs and beds were waiting for more children to arrive.

"At first," Madre Ayau explained to Lauren, "the community will try to keep the children, but they will come to say, 'We cannot feed so many mouths.' They will eventually come here, to the orphanage, after the government shelters can't deal with them."

Madre Ayau said that the government shelters were far more institutional than homes like hers run by the church and by private agencies.

"We're professional beggars," she said of the orphanage, which cost half a million dollars a year to run. It was a constant struggle to fund even the facility's most basic needs. "We don't have a lot of money, but we have a lot of children."

On an afternoon when Lauren was there, she was with the children when they prayed and sang together at a religious service. Later, the boys played soccer while the girls climbed on a jungle gym before gathering for a dinner of rice and *frijoles fritos*, black bean paste spread on bread.

Madre Ayau introduced Lauren to Astrid, a twelve-year-old girl, and her seven-year-old brother, Jember, who were barely surviving on the streets with their mother—a pickpocket who made her children part of her scheme—before arriving at the orphanage six years ago.

"I would like a home for my brother and for me," Astrid confessed at dinner.

Madre Ayau said, "This is the wish of many here, and it will only be compounded with the onslaught of new orphans. It's a never-ending story."

The storm instantly created a major crisis in the country's already overburdened child welfare system, which estimated that upward of 1,200 new orphans were added to the many thousands in the country who were already living in orphanages or on the streets. Throughout Guatemala, between 10,000 and 25,000 orphans literally had nowhere to go. Legal adoption in the country accounted for only 3,500 children per year, most going to the United States, and not all of them orphans. This left a large number of orphans no one even knew about and who many feared would become victims of child trafficking and sexual exploitation. Aside from the few orphans in the care of Madre Ayau and others like her, most of the country's orphaned children were completely unprotected.

Guatemala's newest orphans also faced widespread illnesses such as cholera, dysentery, and hepatitis because of unclean drinking water and the close quarters at shelters.

Lauren went further with her story, exploring the psychological damage to children who had lost their parents in such a violent manner. She spoke with a Red Cross surgeon who confirmed that many of them would be in need of a significant amount of counseling, which of course would not be available to them. Many were reported to have stopped speaking completely; some just stared blankly. There was little for them to do. They had no toys, so they would play with empty medicine dispensers or water bottles.

These scenes, like so many others Lauren witnessed on the trip, were disturbing and tragic. They also need to be documented, and Lauren captured them with her camera as well as with her writing. For that story at least, Lauren *was* a foreign correspondent.

3

Before leaving Guatemala, Lauren and Dina did manage to spend some time together and have fun. They visited Coban, a small town in the northern highlands. It was in a province called Alta Verapaz, which means "true peace" in Spanish. Lauren had done her research, as usual, and had decided that it was a place she had to see. She had been to a number of other Guatemalan tourist towns, but this one was different. It was not as well known, but it had some very beautiful features. The ecosystem there is known as *bosque nuboso*, translated as "cloud forest." It is a type of evergreen mountain forest found in tropical areas, where local conditions cause cloud and mist to form in close contact with the forest vegetation. One of their most obvious features is an abundance of mosses, ferns, orchids, and other similar plants on every tree and rock surface. It also contains the habitat of Guatemala's national bird, the quetzal.

From the army helicopter, Lauren had seen a place called Semuc

Champey, which shimmered with natural pools and waterfalls. Depending on the season, the water can be emerald green or aquamarine—Lauren's birthstone. So she had to go there.

It was a harrowing four-hour drive to Coban from the city, depending on just how bad the conditions of the dirt road were at any given time. It was another four hours over even more treacherous roads to Champey. Dina's husband drove his Suburban. It was a large and capable enough vehicle, but it was no less hazardous as it had to navigate narrow, winding dirt paths where you could only wonder what would happen if another vehicle happened to be coming along in the other direction at the same time. But they managed to reach their destination safely, and it was even more beautiful on the ground than it had been from the air. Lauren stood in front of gleaming mirrors of still, crystalline water fed by magnificent waterfalls cascading down onto the rocks below with all the force of nature. They all marveled at the sight. Lauren took a number of photographs, but they could not do it justice.

The trip back home was torture. It seemed longer and harder, but all the bumps and holes in the road could not shake the smile off Lauren's face, so for Dina it was all worth it. Her husband, however, vowed that he would never go back there again, no matter what.

At the beginning of her trip, the first thing Lauren had wanted to do after Dina picked her up was go to San Judas Tadeo church. The apostle-saint Jude Thaddeus is the "Miraculous Saint," the Catholic patron saint of lost causes and "cases despaired of." Saint Jude is one whose aid is sought when all hope is lost, especially in grave health matters and life-and-death situations. Lauren had taken to wearing a gold medal with an image of Saint Jude around her neck and she prayed to him with blazing faith. She wanted to see the church, so Dina took her. Inside, Lauren knelt in front of a statue of the saint and prayed. Dina joined her and prayed with all her heart, too.

The following year, on September 9, 2006, when Fotofoto Gallery in Huntington, New York, exhibited the photographs that Lauren had taken of the stricken country and its people, she donated all the proceeds from her photo essay, *The Women of Guatemala: Through the Lens, Lauren Terrazzano*, to two charities, a national advocacy group that benefits children called Circle of Friends and a Guatemalan hospital project. Lauren wanted to do something to help build a hospital in an area of Guatemala where there was none.

Before her death on May 15, 2007, she asked that people donate to the Lung Cancer Alliance and to the Obras Sociales del Hermano Pedro, a medical organization in La Antiqua, Guatemala, dedicated to caring for orphaned children, the poor, and the mentally and/or physically incapacitated homeless people of that country.

4

Maureen (Festa) Sergi first met Lauren when they were both incoming freshman at Boston University. They spent two years together on the seventh floor of the Towers. As noted earlier, the International Floor at the Towers was a melting pot of sorts, a place where undergraduates representing a multitude of different nationalities all lived together. Although it was called the International Floor, anyone could live there. Like Lauren, Maureen wanted to live on the International Floor because she was interested in meeting people who came from other parts of the world and learning about different lifestyles and cultures.

The girls had a lot of other things in common as well. Maureen had grown up on the north shore of Boston, in the Merrimack Valley, so they basically came from the same place and had similar backgrounds. Their grandparents were hardworking Italian immigrants with the same values and goals of wanting a better, more prosperous life for their children and grandchildren.

The first thing about Lauren that caught Maureen's attention was her hair, which was huge even by 1986 standards. Because Lauren was such a tiny person with an enormous head of hair, it always seemed to Maureen that she was hiding behind it. She would peer out from behind her chestnut brown locks, and those who did not know her better might have mistaken her as shy and timid, like a frightened rabbit. To Maureen, however, Lauren's behavior was more like a tiger that was hunkered down in the brush, watching and waiting before it strikes. As any of her friends could attest, her headstrong personality was easily evoked. If she were challenged over something she believed in, look out. Nothing could stop her.

Maureen remembers one summer between semesters when Lauren had planned to meet Maureen and her boyfriend in the North End of Boston, where there was the big Italian Feast that weekend. The couple had been waiting a long time for Lauren, who was coming down on the T, the city's commuter rail. Maureen wondered what was keeping her, and she was starting to worry when Lauren suddenly arrived.

"Sorry I'm late," Lauren said. "Had a little problem on the train."

"Was there a breakdown?" Maureen asked.

"No, some asshole tried to steal my purse."

Maureen was instantly shocked and concerned, then looked down and saw that Lauren still had her purse. "Are you okay? What happened?" she asked.

Lauren explained how the would-be robber made a grab for her purse. As he tried to snatch it away from her, however, she held on firmly and started yelling and swearing at the thief, who quickly released the purse and fled the scene empty-handed.

Maureen had to laugh, thinking, *I guess he didn't see the crouching tiger hiding behind the '80s hair.*

The two girls remained friends throughout college, even after they both moved out of the Towers after their sophomore year, Lauren into another dormitory and Maureen off campus. Since Maureen was in the liberal arts curriculum and Lauren was in communications, they did not have any classes together. Maureen was aware of what Lauren was writing in the *Daily Free Press*, BU's independent student newspaper. She read a lot of what Lauren wrote in those years and was impressed that her friend had become a news stringer for United Press International (UPI) while still in college. She wrote stories for the local and national print/broadcast wires, covered spot stories, and was eventually promoted to paid stringer, reporting news associated with Boston University. During the summer before her senior year, Lauren interned under Jeremy Crockford, then the State House Bureau Chief at the *Patriot Ledger* in Quincy, Massachusetts. She covered breaking political news at the State House and also wrote police and community news as well as obituaries.

In later years, Maureen and Lauren saw each other less and less and talked only infrequently. The last time they were together was shortly before Lauren's diagnosis. They had gone out for dinner in New York, meeting at a restaurant in Hell's Kitchen. Lauren was in a good place and content with her life. She loved being a journalist with *Newsday* and was thoroughly enjoying the opportunity she had teaching at Columbia. Over the barbequed food they shared, they talked about everything and caught up on each other's lives.

But Maureen never knew that Lauren got sick and was fighting for her life for nearly three years. She learned that Lauren had passed away only after her mother read about it in the paper and mentioned it to her. Maureen could hardly believe it, even after she found Lauren's "Life, with Cancer" column and went back and read each one.

It made Maureen recall something about Lauren that she had never really thought about before. Maureen had cancer when she was a kid. At the age of thirteen, she was diagnosed with Hodgkin's disease. While she was in college the disease was in remission, but when she was younger she lived in constant fear that it was going to come back and she was going to die. It was something that Maureen talked about often and openly with Lauren, who listened and asked lots of questions. She was very comforting and sympathetic. This was not only what made Lauren a great journalist, it was part of what made her a great friend. Maureen would miss her.

5

It was a couple weeks after the downing of Swissair Flight 111 in the waters off Nova Scotia on September 2, 1998. Lauren had been planning to attend the Journalism & Women Symposium (JAWS) with Monica that fall. It was an event they had both been looking forward to for a long time, but Lauren almost did not go because she was covering the plane crash for *Newsday*. She managed to make it, however, and even though it was an abbreviated stay, she provided a memory that will be remembered for a long time by everyone who was in the newsroom when they returned.

Each year JAWS attracts female reporters, journalism educators, and researchers from across the country and around the world to participate in a series of conferences, lectures, and workshops intended to be one part professional empowerment and growth convention and an equal part personal retreat. The symposium is held every fall in a typically secluded (and always beautiful) locale somewhere in the United States. They never have it in the same place twice, and this time it was in Jackson, Wyoming, along the Snake River in the valley of the Teton Range. It was a place too special for Lauren to pass up visiting, so she took advantage of the opportunity. For millions of tourists, Jackson is not only the gateway to Grand Teton National Park, but Yellowstone National Park as well.

Five female reporters from *Newsday* made the pilgrimage, including Lauren, Monica, and Valerie Kellogg. One afternoon after the conclusion of a lecture, several of the women decided to go out on a hiking expedition into the foothills of the Teton Range of the Rocky Mountains.

For the group of city girls, the countryside was a breathtaking sight to behold, with the vastness of the valley behind them and nature's skyscrapers soaring up in front of them. The women were mostly quiet as they trekked slowly through the lowland mountain region. However, Lauren cautioned the group that they needed to be making more noise in case they unexpectedly came across a bear. She informed them of the danger of startling a bear and said that it was better to make noise that would alert the animal to their presence and frighten it away. At first it was amusing, as Lauren insisted that they all scream and yell out loud as they continued along. At one point Lauren led the group in choruses of "My Favorite Things," "So Long, Farewell," and other songs from *The Sound of Music*, one of her all-time favorite movies.

After a while, some in the group grew weary of this and became disenchanted with Lauren's self-proclaimed wilderness and survival expertise. She did have quite a bit of experience in matters of nature and wildlife, having gone on hiking and camping excursions with her husband, Peter, in a variety of settings, including upstate New York as well as Colorado and Europe and in Hawaii on their honeymoon. Once, she even wrote an article for *Newsday* on trout fishing. But Lauren being the youngest in the group and telling everyone what to do soon began to wear on the other city girls, and eventually one of them told Lauren, only half-jokingly, "Why don't you just shut up? Part of the reason we came up here is to see the wild animals. We don't want to scare them away."

"Oh, no," Lauren insisted. "You don't want to run into a bear or any other wild animal up here at close range."

Everyone laughed—everyone except Lauren. "It's not funny," she said. "It's not funny at all." The other girls only laughed harder at Lauren's expense.

As they turned around to make their way back to the lodge, the group began to splinter, walking individually and several paces apart. When Monica caught up with Lauren, she could see that her friend's serious mood had taken a turn to the morose. She was melancholy and seemed introspective. At one point she broke down and cried, reflecting on some of the tragedies she'd covered, recalling things she had seen, images that included children's dolls and baby carriages being fished out of the water after the crash of TWA Flight 800. She asked Monica how God could allow such terrible things to happen to people.

Monica was taken aback. She had never heard Lauren speak this way. Her friend was clearly distraught, and Monica tried to ease her mind, but she was unreachable. Nothing Monica said seemed to help.

Then all of a sudden Lauren stopped and grabbed Monica by the arm.

"Stay very still," she said.

"Why, what's going on?"

"There's a bear. He's right over there."

"Come on," Monica said dismissively. She thought Lauren was teasing her because of what went on earlier and because Lauren knew how deathly afraid Monica was of bears.

"No, it's true," Lauren told her. "I'm going to tell you what we're going to do."

The others in the group were further ahead on the trail, but they soon noticed that Lauren and Monica had fallen behind. They stopped and waited for the two of them to catch up.

Monica still did not see the bear and started walking to rejoin the group. Then Lauren pointed out where the bear was and Monica froze when she saw the animal. It was about thirty feet away, obscured behind some brush. It appeared to be looking back at them casually.

Instinctively, Monica wanted to run, and she took a couple of steps before Lauren stopped her.

"You can't do that," Lauren said. "Bears run real fast. If they see you running they'll think you're prey and go after you."

Lauren instructed Monica to remain calm and not to run or make any sudden movements. "And make yourself look as big as possible."

"What?"

"Stand on your tiptoes, spread your arms out to your sides, anything to make yourself appear more threatening."

Monica was petrified. She did exactly what Lauren did. A few minutes earlier Monica had been laughing at her, and now Lauren was Les Stroud, Survivorman.

"Bears have bad eyesight," Lauren said, "and might mistake you for a larger animal."

Lauren told Monica to remain calm and to speak in a loud, reassuring voice. With her arms raised high above her head and spread wide, she began moving toward the bear and speaking in a slow, comforting baritone voice. "Hello, Mr. Bear. How are you? Everything is going to be just fine, Mr. Bear. We're not going to hurt you."

"Have you lost your mind, Lauren? What are you doing?"

"This is what you're supposed to do. Come on and do it with me."

Lauren continued in the direction of the bear, which was now staring directly at her.

"Hello, Mr. Bear," she continued. "Don't be afraid, Mr. Bear." And as she got closer, incredibly, the bear started to wander off in the opposite direction. Monica could not believe it worked.

When the bear was safely out of sight behind an outcropping of rock, the two women hightailed it out of there, joining the rest of their group and double-timing it back to the hotel.

From then on, whenever Lauren wanted to get Monica to do something for her, she would always joke about how she'd saved her life that day. But just as Lauren would never let Monica forget it, Lauren's friends and colleagues in the newsroom would never let her live it down either. As more people at *Newsday* heard about the incident, it became a source of levity and lighthearted teasing for some time afterward. It would not be uncommon for fellow reporters at the newspaper to greet Lauren or Monica when they walked in by raising up their arms and chanting, "Hello, Mr. Bear. How are you?"

Eight

Measureless Gratitude to Unsung Caregivers

I haven't checked the Hallmark aisle recently, but it raised the question of how we recognize the thousands of people who are fighting alongside us in the cancer war—or in any bout with a serious injury or chronic illness.

Society calls them informal "caregivers." I call them daily miracle workers who plod along with a quiet humanity that often gets overlooked.

Nurses will occasionally get a tray of cookies from grateful patients at the end of a particularly civilized hospital stay or when they manage to get the IV into your arm on the first try. And doctors are frequently the recipients of a patient or family's eternal gratitude or a bottle of fine cognac.

But the fact is, with Thanksgiving approaching, it's hard to find the appropriate way to thank the unsung warriors who make your life easier.

That would be the spouse who makes midnight ginger ale runs. Or who is with you at every scary medical appointment, in a sterile examining room where time is marked by the tick of a wristwatch or an anxiously beating heart.

There doesn't seem to be a suitable way to acknowledge the friends who will take your frantic phone calls past midnight, wash your dishes without even being asked, bear the brunt of your descent into rage when your hair starts to fall out, or are willing to take off with you on a whim, even overseas, just because you need to get away.

And let's not forget mothers, fathers, sisters or brothers forced to watch with an ugly, helpless fear as their child or sibling goes through the hell that is cancer treatment. There is no balloon bouquet or greeting card for their pain.

Yet, these are the people who are expected to go on with life without missing a beat. They go to work each day and still manage to take care of us, performing a delicate balancing act as they neglect their own emotional or physical needs. And after the war is over, for better or worse, they are also left with scars.

—From *Newsday*, "Life, with Cancer," November 21, 2006, "Measureless Gratitude to Unsung Caregivers," by Lauren Terrazzano

1

In late 1999 and early 2000 Monica began to notice that Lauren started to complain about being exhausted all the time and having frequent headaches. At first Monica attributed it to the hectic pace Lauren had set for herself as a journalist since she started at *Newsday*. She had run nonstop from the beginning. It was also around this time that Monica became very concerned for Lauren's health because she noticed an obvious loss in her friend's weight.

The one criticism of Lauren that Monica had was how demanding she was of herself at work and how hard she pushed herself, to the point of excess. Monica would see her friend running herself ragged and felt she had to say something. On far too many occasions to count, she would caution Lauren to take it easy. Monica would remind her that she was still young.

"It takes time," was a phrase Monica repeated ad nauseum to Lauren over the course of several months during that time. The point she wanted to make was that they were in a very competitive field and a journalist's reputation is not made overnight. She repeatedly tried to convince Lauren to take some time off, do something fun with her husband, go camping, hiking, just enjoy herself. But Lauren was already doing exactly what she loved. Reporting.

Looking back later, Monica feels that it was almost as if Lauren knew that she did not have a long time on earth and wanted to accomplish everything she could while she still had the chance. She had such clear goals in mind of where she wanted to be, and she was not going to compromise those goals.

As with all good friends, Monica and Lauren had their share of disagreements, but Lauren's management of her own well-being became the cause of one of the few serious fights the two of them ever had. The final straw came when Lauren confessed to Monica, completely out of the blue, that she was not happy. It was not so much what she said as the way she said it that unnerved Monica. Lauren's voice and demeanor, she said, were filled with utter despair and hopelessness. She started talking about things that had never come up in their talks before. Monica could only listen as Lauren continued to speak. It became more of a monologue than a conversation. Monica thought it was like reading her friend's diary.

Lauren also retraced some of the missteps in her life, reflecting on her failed marriage to Peter and about how she may have rushed into it because she wanted to make her mother happy.

"I worry about them," she told Monica. "I'm their only child." Monica knew how close Lauren was to us and how she sometimes became a little overprotective of her mother and me. Lauren went on further, telling Monica that she loved us, but she also felt a strong responsibility for us as well. She wanted to make sure nothing ever happened to us, that we didn't worry and that we were happy. She told Monica that she didn't want to let us down.

"I don't know what to do," Lauren said finally, in resignation.

Then Lauren admitted to her friend that she did not know the meaning of life, and that was when Monica became most concerned.

"Lauren, have you talked to anyone else about this?"

Lauren shook her head.

"You have to talk to someone," Monica said. "Your parents at least?"

"No," Lauren snapped.

"It'll help you."

"I don't want them knowing. Don't you tell anyone."

She didn't know what Lauren might do, but Monica knew that she had to do something. She didn't think anything she said would get through to Lauren in the current state of mind her friend was in. Monica realized she had to go to a third party. She didn't think Lauren would ever forgive her if she went to Ginny and me, knowing how protective she was of us. She thought of Peter next. With their marriage unraveling (the couple had recently separated), it was not an ideal time for a personal intervention. Monica, however, thought it was necessary. She also thought that their friendship was strong enough to handle that.

Monica had not been afforded very many opportunities to inter-act with Peter over the years, and Lauren did not tell her much about their relationship, but Monica decided to confide in Peter and express her very serious concerns about Lauren to him.

Monica told Peter everything, and he became alarmed, agreeing that Lauren's behavior was troubling and something needed to be done. He felt compelled to help, and he was grateful to Monica for letting him know. He promised he would have a talk with Lauren. The next time he saw her he brought it up, but when Lauren learned that it was Monica's mediation that had prompted his unexpected visit and sudden interest in her welfare, she became very upset. She did not appreciate the fact that they had been talking about her "behind her back," but much of her ire was directed at Monica for talking to Peter about something that she had spoken to her about in confidence. Lauren reacted sternly, chastising Monica for what she considered her betrayal. Monica tried to explain that it was only with her best interests in mind that she had reached out to Peter with the hope that he might be able help, but it was to no avail. Lauren withdrew, alienating herself from Monica, and for a time they did not speak. No more daily phone calls. At work they barely acknowledged each other. This went on for almost six months. It was a difficult time for the friends, and as they both got busy with their work, Lauren's marriage with Peter did come to an end.

Working at the same newspaper and having a lot of the same friends, Lauren and Monica were never really apart, at least physically, and that made it easier for them to patch things up, which they eventually did one day when Lauren approached Monica, who heard Lauren's familiar, "Hey, Cruella."

Monica looked around smiling, knowing Lauren was talking to her.

"You want to be friends again?" Lauren asked.

"Sure."

"Good," Lauren said, and as she was turning to leave she added, "I have a lot to do. I'll call you tonight, BMQ."

"Okay, LT Supremo. Talk to you later."

After that, it was as if the falling out had never happened, and it was something they never talked about again. Lauren disliked conflict. If there was a chance to achieve harmony in any way, she would seek it out.

2

It wasn't until late 1999 that I heard the name Al Baker for the first time. Lauren had never mentioned him as far as I can recall. I didn't know who he was, and I didn't know that he also a journalist with *Newsday*. Late that summer, the newspaper sent Lauren up to Albany to cover State House news. They put her up in a leased apartment, and she was supposed to be up there for three months. She didn't mind the assignment. It would give her some experience with political journalism, and someone else would take her place after three months.

Right near the end of her stint in Albany, I called her like I usually did just about every day if she didn't call us. A man picked up the apartment phone, which startled me for a moment. He quickly introduced himself as Al Baker, a reporter with *Newsday*, and explained that he was taking over the State House coverage after Lauren. I wished him luck and asked him to let Lauren know that I called. "I hope everything works out for you," I told him.

I don't know exactly when they began seeing each other. Lauren didn't talk a lot about him, at least not to me. She mentioned something about him to her mother first, and that's how I found out they were dating. He was divorced with no children. In early 2000 he started working for the *New York Times*, the main competitor of *Newsday*.

Ginny visited Lauren in New York about once every two months without me. She would take the train down for some mother-daughter time; they'd go shopping and out to eat. One weekend Lauren invited her mother to New York to meet Al. They went out for dinner together, and from what I gathered, everyone had a pleasant time.

"He's a big teddy bear," Lauren said of Al. When Lauren asked her mother what she thought of Al, Ginny didn't say what she actually thought. She told me later that there was something about the man that she just didn't trust, but it wasn't the kind of thing she would say about a man that her daughter liked enough to arrange to have them meet. Ginny was smart enough to know that it wouldn't do anybody any good. It would only cause a problem, an argument perhaps, or worse, Ginny thought—alienate her daughter.

The following morning, Al met the ladies for breakfast and presented Ginny with a bouquet of flowers. Ginny appreciated the gesture. She thanked him, and on the train ride back, Ginny was carrying the flowers with her when a passenger beside her complained, "Some people are allergic to those, you know." Much later when she told me that story, I had to laugh.

Lauren and Al dated on and off for a while, and we always knew when they were not together. When Lauren would visit us and she was in a bad mood, we knew it probably had to do with Al. Ginny would ask what was going on between them and Lauren would confide that they had broken up again. When pressed about it, invariably Lauren's response would be, "I don't want to talk about it."

One issue we knew might be a source of conflict was Lauren's competitiveness. She never liked to divulge the details of any investigative story she was working on, even to Al. Maybe especially to him, since he was now a reporter for the competition, the *New York Times*.

3

Tomoeh Tse joined the *Newsday* staff in the spring of 2003. Though she came in with some experience, having worked at a number of different newspapers over the previous few years, she was still young and impressionable. She had known she wanted to be a journalist from an early age and set out on that career path. She was born and raised in Japan, where journalists were traditionally little more than instruments of the government, so she endeavored to make her way to the United States as soon as possible. She transferred to Stanford University to study journalism and learn the craft. She wrote for the school paper, and after graduation she interned at several newspapers around the country before landing her first staff writing position in Cleveland with the *Cleveland Plain Dealer*, the largest newspaper in Ohio. Desiring to work in New York, where her boyfriend (and future husband) worked as a graphic artist for the *New York Times*, she sent her resume to every newspaper publisher in the city. When an offer came back from *Newsday* she jumped at it.

Tomoeh was well aware of Lauren's stature and ability as a writer before she started at *Newsday*. As far back as 2000, when Tomoeh was writing for the *Plain Dealer*, Lauren's stories always impressed her. She was very excited just to be working at the same paper as Lauren. One year Tomoeh had been a nominee for a Livingston award, a national honor issued to media professionals under thirty-five for local, national, and international reporting. The Livingston award differs from others such as the Peabody and the Pulitzer prize in that the entries in each category are judged against one another, and as a consequence are widely regarded as the most prestigious and competitive award that a young journalist can receive. Tomoeh had been honored to see her name listed alongside Lauren's when both of them were named among the cofinalists for the award. Being considered a journalistic peer alongside Lauren was more exciting to Tomoeh than the award itself, so when she arrived at *Newsday* and found her desk situated just in front of Lauren's space with Sylvia Adcock's desk between them, she was somewhat starstruck.

Lauren was hard at work on the assisted-living project, so Tomoeh only got glimpses of her as she moved back and forth between the investigative room to her other desk in the newsroom. Tomoeh hoped she might be able to learn from Lauren someday, and in time the two women would indeed come into closer contact.

Upon first meeting Lauren, Tomoeh expected that a successful, motivated, New York journalist like Lauren would be more cynical and even more sophisticated, but she found Lauren to be as grounded and as down-to-earth as anyone she had ever known. Tomoeh was delighted and surprised by how friendly Lauren was, and she was delighted to get to know her for who she really was.

If anything, Tomoeh thought Lauren should have been more impressed with herself. It was bewildering how insecure she could be at times about her writing. Tomoeh noticed that Lauren was always questioning if what she had written was any good or not. It was more than surprising, and sometimes Tomoeh struggled to convince her. Her stories always came out well, and if it was her insecurity that was pushing her and motivating her to be better, there was no arguing with the results. She never rested on her laurels, and instead worked longer and harder on a project. It didn't seem that Lauren even heard the praise that Tomoeh and others heaped upon her, and she certainly didn't realize how much Tomoeh admired her. Tomoeh was just glad that Lauren was comfortable enough to open up to her the way she did about her insecurities. For all that, she was still a confident and aggressive journalist, one of the best at what she did; she just was not arrogant about her writing the way some journalists could be.

Since Tomoeh was living on the West Side and Lauren was on the upper West Side of Manhattan, it was convenient for Tomoeh to carpool with Lauren and Dawn McKeen. It was during those drives out to Long Island that Tomoeh really got to know Lauren. The first thing Lauren taught her was the various shortcuts through the city streets that could knock off up to twenty minutes of the usual hour and a half one-way trip.

Tomoeh expected that Lauren would be listening to National Public Radio or to a classical music station in the car and was amazed by the sappy music stations that Lauren typically tuned into. She was further surprised by the various topics of conversation that came up. Tomoeh, who had anticipated a more sophisticated choice of music, would have figured that the en route discussions would have been similarly urbane. She didn't think she would have anything to contribute other than sitting quietly and nodding, but the others chatted about silly or everyday things. One of the first things Lauren talked about with Tomoeh was how she wanted to see the recently released Julia Roberts movie, *Mona Lisa Smile*, which was coming out soon. Tomoeh loved Julia Roberts, too, and when Lauren told her that the

actress had actually been studying journalism herself before getting into films, the two women seemed to bond almost instantly.
The nearly ten-year difference in age helped facilitate an older sister–younger sister relationship between them. Lauren began calling
Tomoeh "Froggy," or sometimes "Little Froggy," because Lauren said
that Tomoeh sounded like a frog one day when she started to whine
about something, and the nickname stuck. After that, naturally,
everyone in Lauren's circle started calling Tomeoh "Froggy" except
for Monica, who called her "Frogolina" instead.

The following year, when Lauren was sick but had the strength to
go to the movies for the first time in a while, she chose *Bridget Jones:
The Edge of Reason*. It was a girly romantic comedy, but those were
just the kinds of sappy movies—like her music—that Lauren liked.

4

In the summer of 2004, Lauren was not well. It was obvious to
Monica that her friend was not quite herself, that she was suffering from some kind of malaise that was really too vague to ascribe to
anything specific.

Lauren was not seeing anyone at that time. Her relationship with
Al Baker had been running hot and cold for the past few years, and
they had broken up about eight months earlier—and it seemed to
be for good this time. That wasn't what was bothering her, however.
Something just wasn't right physically. The sense that something
was wrong manifested itself primarily in an overwhelming fatigue
that she could not shake. This was not a sudden condition; it had

been going on for quite some time, but only now was it starting to catch up with her enough so that she noticed. She had to practically drag herself out of bed each morning, and she began to find that she was not able to rebound during the course of the day. She remained exhausted until she went to bed at night.

This was a difficult time in Lauren's life. She was working as hard as ever and driving to Boston almost every weekend to be with her mom, who had begun experiencing kidney problems. It was a hectic pace, and because of this Lauren probably didn't take what her body was telling her as seriously as she should have.

It was just before the Fourth of July, when Lauren and Monica were talking at work, that Lauren confided in her friend about her constant exhaustion. She admitted that she had never been so tired in her life.

At first, Monica told me later, she was in denial as well. She wanted to believe that her friend was burning the candle at both ends and just needed some time off to relax. The assisted-living series had taken a lot out of her, and now that it was running in the paper, Monica suggested to Lauren that she slow down a little.

"You're right," Lauren said simply.

"Seriously, you should take some vacation time. Go away somewhere. If I have to go with you to make sure of it, I will."

"Okay. You're on. But I pick where we go."

"You got it," Monica said. "So, do you have plans for the holiday weekend? Are you going home to see your parents?"

"No. I'll be in the city. I have some things I need to finish up at work." Lauren saw the way Monica was looking at her then added, "Before I go on vacation."

"Hey," Monica said, "why don't you stop by? We'll be home all weekend. You could relax by the pool, unwind."

"Yeah. That sounds good. Count on it, Cruella."

"Great. I'll see you this weekend."

But Monica never heard from Lauren that weekend. She did not stop by as she said she would, and when Monica tried calling her she did not pick up the phone, which was not like her if she was at home. The holiday weekend came and went, and when Monica saw Lauren at work the following week, Monica asked what happened.

Lauren said that she just got too tired, and she thought she was experiencing anxiety attacks.

"Anxiety!" Monica said. "What made you think it was anxiety?"

"Well, I went to the emergency room the other day because I couldn't breathe. I was panting and having a hard time catching my breath."

"Oh my God, Lauren! Why didn't you call me?"

"I didn't want to bother you on a holiday."

"You call for lot lesser things than that. We weren't doing anything this weekend. I told you. You could have at least called."

"It was probably nothing."

"What do you mean? What did the doctors say?"

Lauren said that she had gone to the ER, waited there for more than an hour, and then just left because she hadn't been seen. "There were too many people and it was too busy there," Lauren said. "It's probably nothing anyway."

Monica was deeply worried. "No, Lauren," she said. "That's not normal. You shouldn't be having anxiety attacks."

"I was probably just freaking out because of what's going on with my mother," Lauren said.

"No," Monica said, unconvinced. "You need to make an appointment with your doctor to try to find out exactly what's going on. You need to do it right away, Lauren. You can't just blow it off. This is your health."

"Okay. I'll call."

"I mean it, Lauren. Promise me."

"I promise. Honest."

Lauren didn't just agree with Monica to put the matter behind her. She truly intended to make an appointment with her doctor to find out what was wrong, but all her focus remained on her concern for Ginny, who had begun experiencing debilitating pain that would later be diagnosed as part of a serious kidney disorder. Lauren felt that her own health issue was far less significant, more of a distraction than an inconvenience, in light of her mother's condition. Anyway, besides the fatigue, she felt fine.

She was too busy to be sick.

5

The relationship between Sylvia Adcock and Lauren was based on mutual interests and friends. They may not have been finishing each other's sentences, but they were like-minded. One of the things they had in common was that they were both admitted hypochondriacs. For no reason that either of them could fully understand, they would occasionally go online and look up various diseases. Invariably, they would determine that they were experiencing a symptom or two of a particular disease before pronouncing that they might be suffering from the very same affliction. They would always end up laughing uncomfortably, having given themselves a good scare, but they knew they were all right. Their dark humor was so much whistling past the graveyard. Still, such issues of human mortality seemed to be something that concerned them both. Perhaps it was the years they'd spent as journalists, reporting on all sorts of horrific accidents and environmental hazards that other people had experienced that caused the two women to think about their own mortality from time to time.

The day Lauren first mentioned the swollen vein on her arm, however, Sylvia was not laughing. She could clearly see that the upper part of Lauren's right arm was noticeably larger than the other.

"Look at this," Lauren told Sylvia, indicating her swollen arm. "This is crazy. How can I have one arm bigger than the other? I'm going to become one of those Italian grandmothers with the big flabby arm."

Lauren smiled, but Sylvia became concerned. She thought she recognized a certain discomfort lurking behind the smile on Lauren's face. Sylvia wondered what it could be, but did not say anything to Lauren.

Very much on their minds was a friend and coworker at *Newsday* who had died suddenly as the result of a blood clot at the age of forty. Now they were both thinking the same thing as they looked at the unusual swelling.

"You need to get that looked at," Sylvia said.

"I'll keep an eye on it," Lauren said dismissively. She felt—or wanted to believe—that it was much more likely to be nothing, and that they were overreacting.

By this time, Lauren's other friends and coworkers began to notice this physical anomaly as well. Among them was Tomoeh, who after noticing Lauren's swollen arm also pushed her to go to the doctor for a checkup.

6

On August 21, 2004, Lauren came home to see us for the weekend. During this trip, she spent a lot of time with her childhood friend Leah.

Although the girls had gone through brief periods where they did not see a lot of each other, they had long since reconnected. While Lauren was away at college, Leah commuted to local Merrimack College in nearby Andover. During that time, Lauren didn't come home many weekends, wanting to explore (after her tumultuous first semester) the whole Boston University experience. After Lauren graduated and moved to New York, the girls resumed their previous close friendship. Leah visited New York often, shopping with Lauren, going out to eat, and having girls' nights out. The two girls went on vacations together, including a memorable 1991 trip to Italy where they were almost arrested because they got on a bus without purchasing a ticket. The bus inspector tried to remove them at the next stop and turn them over to the authorities, but Lauren talked her way out of trouble, conversing with the man in Italian. He let them stay on the bus and the two girls later laughed about the episode, but at the time

Leah was worried. She thought they were going to wind up in some Italian jail where no one would ever hear from them again. Instead, they went on to enjoy the rest of their time in Rome, Venice, and Naples. Everyone they met was very friendly, and naturally Lauren and Leah caught the attention of a few young Italian men. When they met two guys who told them they would come to visit them in the United States sometime, neither of them thought that it would ever really happen. But then a month later the two Italian guys showed up at both their doors. Leah could not believe it. Fortunately, the guys had friends in New York and in northern New England.

Later, as Lauren's marriage to Peter started to deteriorate, she and Leah began to drift apart again. Around the same time, Leah was busy getting her doctoral degree at the University of Maryland. Lauren visited her there once, but they didn't see each other much. After Lauren's divorce, however, they resumed their friendship as it was before.

On that weekend in August 2004, Lauren was feeling pretty down. Looking for a lift, she called Leah and suggested they go to an amusement park. Leah was all for it, and off they went to Canobie Lake Park in Salem, New Hampshire. They went on the dodgem cars, the antique carousel, rode around the park on the Canobie Express, and drove the antique cars. They got some strange looks from people when they went on a few of the kiddie rides, but they had a great time. It was a beautiful day and Lauren was wearing a short-sleeve shirt, which called attention not only to the inflammation in her right arm, but also to what appeared at first to be a bruise.

"What happened to your arm?" Leah asked at one point.

"Yeah," Lauren said, and pulled her sleeve up further so Leah could get a better look at it. "What do you think about this?"

Leah saw clearly that what she thought was a bruise was actually a bluish-purple blood vessel bulging prominently from Lauren's upper arm near her shoulder. "That looks weird," she said.

"I must have banged it on something," Lauren said. "I don't remember doing it. It doesn't seem to be going away. I know I should probably get it looked at."

"Yeah," Leah agreed. "I would. Does it hurt?"

"Nah," Lauren said and rolled her sleeve back down, her thoughts on something else entirely.

The girls spent the rest of that afternoon at the amusement park then headed home. They were both wiped out and drove most of the way listening to the radio, without talking. Lauren crashed almost as soon as she got home. She had told Leah that she was going to schedule a time for her doctor to look at her arm, and this time she followed through on it. She made an appointment for the following week and she meant to keep it. What she hadn't told Leah was that she had noticed a smaller cluster of tiny veins that had appeared above her right breast sometime in the preceding weeks.

On Thursday, August 26, Monica saw Lauren in the newsroom and noticed the unusual discoloration on her upper right arm. It was raised slightly and looked like a bump. Monica asked Lauren if she had fallen and hurt herself.

"I don't know what happened," Lauren said.

Upon closer inspection, Monica saw the protruding blood vessel and became instantly alarmed.

"Lauren! What is that? How long have you had that?"

"Not long," Lauren said.

"It looks like a vein. Are you going to the doctor? You said you were."

"Yeah, yeah," Lauren said. "I made an appointment. I'm going to St. Luke's tomorrow."

"All right. Make sure you call me. I don't have to work tomorrow. I'm going to be in the city, at Columbia University, so give me a call. Maybe we can get together, have lunch."

"Okay," Lauren said. "I'll call you tomorrow."

"Make sure you call me."

"I will."

The following day, Lauren was searching courthouse records for an investigative piece she was working on about corrupt homeless-shelter operators when she realized that she had a doctor's appointment that afternoon. She had almost forgotten about it, and she immediately put down what she was doing and left for the hospital, knowing it would take some time to make her way across town to St. Luke's-Roosevelt Hospital Center on the West Side.

Nine

Secrets from the
Alternate Universe

I've never understood the people who insist that getting cancer was the best thing that ever happened to them. I could have done without this so-called epiphany in my life. My family and friends could have as well.

Still, the one enlightening thing about it—and this is a stretch—is that getting such a disease offers a certain perspective that often eludes the rest of the world.

We travelers on this road have learned a secret: the value of time. Down to the day. The minute. The second.

We are forced to confront our own mortality every day.

We see the bus coming straight at us, while other people never knew what hit them. So we cram as much life as we can into whatever time there is left, because each doctor's appointment or scan is a dress rehearsal for the bad news we know could ultimately come, as one reader wrote to me recently.

Still, many who have never had a life-threatening experience tend to plod along toward infinity with what I call luxury problems: Worrying about the thread count on their expensive sheets, why they didn't get that raise, or how to get their kid into the right school.

How I long for the days of such worries. How I long to go back to the time when my biggest concern was where my story played in the newspaper, not whether a suspicious dark spot would show up on my CT scan.

This is not to diminish other people's dramas. If you want to exist among the living, you have to acknowledge the rest of the world doesn't know what it's like to wait for the results of a biopsy or to undergo chemotherapy.

Unfortunately, many of us do.

—From *Newsday*, "Life, with Cancer," December 5, 2006,
"Secrets from the Alternate Universe" by Lauren Terrazzano

1

St. Luke's-Roosevelt Hospital Center is an academic affiliate of Columbia University College of Physicians and Surgeons and is actually comprised of two hospital components, St. Luke's Hospital and Roosevelt Hospital.

That afternoon, Lauren visited St. Luke's to be evaluated by a vascular surgeon, Dr. Alan Benvenisty, with whom she had her appointment. She had to wait some time before being seen, but she was feeling pretty good about finally doing what everybody had been telling her she should do for the last month or so. Despite everything leading up this fateful day, Lauren still believed they would run a couple tests, the doctor would give her the old spiel about getting more sleep and exercise, and she would be out of there in plenty of time to have dinner with Monica, who was just across the street at Columbia University.

The first diagnostic test was an ultrasound of her arm. Initially, the vascular surgeon suggested that the problem might be the result of a blot clot. This was followed up by a chest x-ray, which revealed something else entirely.

It identified a mass.

"It could be an infection," Dr. Benvenisty said. He looked at Lauren soberly. "But most likely not."

Lauren knew that a mass meant only one thing. If it wasn't an infection that could be eradicated with a simple round of antibiotics, that all but confirmed it. She didn't want to say it out loud, so she didn't say anything at all.

This wasn't happening, she thought. *He had to be joking.*

Dr. Benvenisty was the director of the renal transplantation program at the hospital and was not a man who would make such a claim without knowing what he was talking about.

Lauren was becoming extremely concerned, but then the doctor called his wife to tell her he would be late coming home, and that was when she became really scared. A precautionary afternoon checkup had turned into a complete battery of tests, and now the specter of a serious health issue raised its head. The thought of cancer was lurking somewhere in her mind, but she wasn't ready to sound that alarm just yet.

Dr. Benvenisty told Lauren that he wanted to have a CT scan, a sophisticated x-ray, performed right away, saying that the imaging it produced would provide a much more accurate picture of what he had detected. Lauren, of course, agreed to have the procedure done.

When asked if she smoked, Lauren responded that she had, though only for a relatively brief time. Over the past six years she had smoked on and off, mostly off. It really was more of a nervous habit than an addiction, developed at the ripe old age of thirty as a result of some personal turmoil in her life, mainly the end of her marriage to Peter. She probably smoked most freely when she was abroad. She traveled frequently, particularly to Italy, where everyone seemed to have a cigarette dangling from their lips. In 2000, she made a pact with a friend at work and they both gave it up for about a year. But on September 11, 2001, when Lauren saw bodies falling from the World Trade Center, before she thought about it she'd rushed out and bought a pack of cigarettes. In the wake of the terror attacks, she could not light up fast enough. Shortly after that, though, she quit again. She picked up the habit and then stopped several more times in the ensuing years. In the fall of 2003 she started up while on an assignment in Spain for *Newsday*.

Dr. Benvenisty didn't think that Lauren should be alone at that time and asked her if there was anyone she wanted him to call to come and be with her.

Lauren was temporarily stymied by the request. She couldn't think for a minute. It seemed so unreal. It was as if she was watching one of her sappy movies and she was waiting to see what was going to happen next.

Lauren was in a near panic when she gave the doctor the name of her closest friend and colleague at *Newsday*, Monica Quintanilla. She watched as he dialed the phone number she gave him.

2

By the time Monica finished up her business in the city for the day and was getting ready to head home, she had yet to hear from Lauren. She had checked her cell phone several times, but there were no calls from Lauren. Monica knew Lauren would have called if she could have, so Monica deduced that Lauren was still at the hospital and was unable to use her phone. Monica had no choice but to drive back to New Jersey. She had a trip to Spain planned and she was leaving in a couple of days. She needed to get a few things at the mall and had promised her nieces that she would pick them up on her way home and take them with her.

She checked the time again. It was after 2:00. Lauren had a one o'clock appointment. A routine exam wouldn't have taken this long, she reasoned, and then she suddenly decided to call Lauren. She tried her home number first. No answer. Then her cell phone. Nothing.

At around 3:30, Monica and the girls were not quite at the mall yet when Monica's phone rang. It was a number Monica did not recognize, but something told her she should answer it.

"Hello," she said.

"Is this Monica?"

"Yes. Who is this?"

"I am Dr. Alan Benvenisty. I'm calling from St. Luke's Hospital. I'm with your friend, Lauren."

"Oh my God! What happened? Is she okay?"

"Well, I ran some tests on her today . . . Can you come to the hospital today?"

"When?" Monica asked.

"Well, right now."

"Sure, sure. What has happened?"

"You really have to come in."

"Can I talk to Lauren?"

"Certainly."

Lauren got on the phone and Monica asked her what was wrong. Lauren told her that the doctor was performing some standard tests to try to determine what was causing the swelling in her arm when an x-ray revealed some spots in her chest. Monica asked to speak to the doctor and questioned him about what he planned to do next. He told her that he wanted to have a CT scan performed. Monica said she needed to take her nieces home first and that it would take her about half an hour to get back into the city from New Jersey. The doctor promised he wouldn't do anything until she got there.

After dropping her nieces off at home, Monica drove straight to

St. Luke's to meet Lauren. They hugged and talked for a while as they waited for Dr. Benvenisty to return. The girls were all very emotional, but Lauren was also strangely serene, Monica thought. At one point, Lauren said in a matter-of-fact way, "I did myself in."

"What are you talking about, Lauren?" Monica asked her.

"I didn't take care of myself."

Monica did not want to approve such a self-indictment and had started to say something to Lauren when Dr. Benvenisty walked into the room and introduced himself. Together, they all went with Lauren to have her CT scan. Dr. Benvenisty personally walked them across the street to the radiology department.

The entire procedure took less than twenty minutes to complete, and while Dr. Benvenisty pored over the results, Lauren did not mince words. "Look, I don't want any bullshit," she said. "Just give it to me straight. Tell me what it is. You have to tell me the truth. I am an only child and my parents mean the world to me. So just tell me because I need to get ready and I need to get my parents ready."

With Monica by Lauren's side, Dr. Benvenisty told her that the test confirmed conclusively what the x-ray had shown. There was a large mass on the right side her chest, pressing directly against her lung. He said that the scan further determined that there were also three smaller masses in the same area, along the lining of her right lung.

"By masses you mean tumors?" Monica asked.

"Yes. That's correct."

Everyone took a deep breath.

"Doctor," Monica began, "what are the chances that these masses are benign?"

He shook his head and told her there was virtually no chance they were nonmalignant.

Lauren was unable to stifle a cry the moment that the doctor made the pronouncement. He told her that the tumor that had attached itself directly on her lung was the most threatening and was probably responsible for the difficulty she had been having catching her breath—it was pressing on her lung. The vascular surgeon also indicated that the mass was almost certainly interfering with the blood flow to her right arm, causing the veins to protrude there.

Lauren asked what needed to be done next. Dr. Benvenisty told her that a biopsy would have to be performed, and he suggested that she meet with a chest specialist to perform the biopsy. This was a detail that was not lost on Lauren. She was aware that Dr. Benvenisty never used the words "lung cancer." In fact, he had never actually said "cancer." However, he had asked her if she smoked. Now, he had asked her to consult a chest specialist—a thoracic surgeon. And a thoracic surgeon meant lung cancer. A biopsy was necessary to determine exactly what type of cancer it was and at what stage.

All these things were going through Lauren's mind when Dr. Benvenisty gave her the name of the oncologist at the hospital and set up an appointment for her the following day. He said that the oncologist would schedule a biopsy and once he got the results he (Dr. Benvenisty) would be able to give her more information.

Lauren did not hear a word he was saying, but fortunately Monica was there to write everything down. Dr. Benvenisty had been very kind and Monica thanked him for all that he had done for Lauren.

Monica took Lauren home, and once there she cried a little bit more. She clearly felt guilty and blamed herself for getting sick, telling Monica once again, "I really did myself in. I didn't take good enough care of myself."

"That's nonsense, Lauren," Monica said. "You didn't do anything wrong."

"What am I going to tell my parents? How can I tell them that their only child has cancer? I can't tell them."

"If you want me to break it to them, Lauren, I'll do it for you."

"No," Lauren cried out. "Promise you won't, Monica. No one can tell them."

It was not at all surprising to Monica that Lauren would be so adamantly opposed to letting us know about her health crisis. She was sure that this was where most of Lauren's guilt emanated from: she would blame herself for causing Ginny and me to worry about her, and that was a great burden for her to bear. But it was not an issue Monica wanted to trouble Lauren with at that time. She knew it would not be a secret for very long, so she assured Lauren that she would not say anything to anyone.

Lauren called Leah, her oldest friend from childhood, and Sylvia, who in some ways had come to see Lauren as a daughter. These were the two people Lauren called first, not her mother and me.

Lauren asked Sylvia to come to her apartment the following day. That morning, too, Leah was on the plane to New York. She wanted to be by Lauren's side during this difficult time, and she arrived from Boston in time to accompany her friend on her initial visit with her oncologist. Monica and Sylvia also went with her to St. Luke's Hospital that Saturday afternoon.

After a brief consultation, the answers Lauren provided the doctor suggested the possibility of lymphoma, with leukemia being ruled out. A biopsy, as Dr. Benvenisty also suggested, would be the only way to know for sure what type of tumor she had.

Lauren was concerned that the procedure might cause the cancer cells to proliferate. She wanted to make absolutely certain that this would not happen and began asking the doctor a series of questions. In the end, she determined that she was not comfortable having the biopsy done at St. Luke's. Lauren had a lot of respect and trust for her friend Dr. Akhtar Ashfaq, a nephrologist and doctor of internal medicine, and decided that she wanted Dr. Ashfaq to oversee the biopsy. He did not perform the procedure himself, but he ensured her that it was done in a timely manner and he would get the results back to her right away. He arranged to have the procedure done the following Thursday at North Shore University Hospital in Manhasset, New York, where he practiced.

After leaving St. Luke's, the girls spent the rest of the afternoon together. They didn't talk much about Lauren's health. They had something to eat and walked around the city in a kind of collective daze. They decided to conclude the day with walk through Central Park. It was hot and sticky right into the evening, making an already uncomfortable day worse. It must have affected Lauren's mood because the way she reacted to a homeless man who approached them surprised everyone. When he told them that he had no job and no food (as he stuck out his hand), Lauren stopped suddenly and confronted him. She looked him directly in the eyes and shouted, "Yeah, well, I have cancer!" Then she turned away and continued walking, leaving the man standing there with his hand still extended. They all saw the irony of this—Lauren had always been someone who helped the downtrodden. Now there she was, practically yelling at a vagrant who was begging for spare change in the park.

3

With Labor Day weekend coming up, Leah decided to stay with Lauren for the entire week, going with her for her biopsy first and then for other appointments she might have coming up. Monica also went with them to North Shore University Hospital for Lauren's biopsy. The procedure went well and was quick. Lauren was told that it shouldn't be long before the results were in and a determination made from the biopsy. Dr. Ashfaq said he would call her as soon as any information was available.

Monica was scheduled to leave for Spain that week, but she told Lauren that she would gladly postpone her trip for another time. Lauren insisted that she go.

"I'm not going to be able enjoy it under these conditions," Monica said.

"You've had this trip planned for a long time. You have to go. I'll be okay. When you return, that's when I'm going to need you most."

Monica acquiesced. She felt a lot better knowing Leah would be staying with Lauren all week.

It was difficult for Lauren to wait for the news. She was a journalist, after all, who was used to going out and getting information. Waiting for it was something completely foreign to her. Even as she went about her business and usual hectic routine, she couldn't stop thinking about the pending results. It was almost as if she didn't want it sneaking up on her, because if it did that would somehow make the results even worse. She called Dr. Ashfaq several times over the course of the next couple days to ask if any confirmation had been made as to the type of cancer they found in the biopsied tissue. Each time he told her that the reports had not come back yet.

Finally, at the end of the second day, Dr. Ashfaq stopped by Lauren's apartment to give her the news in person. She knew immediately why he was there, and she waited for him to say it. He told her quickly.

"It's lung cancer," he said.

They embraced and cried.

"I'm sorry, Lauren."

"What stage is it?" Lauren asked.

"That we don't know just yet. Some further tests have to be performed."

These weren't all the answers she needed and this wasn't what she wanted to hear, but it was what she was expecting. Lauren still wasn't ready to tell her mother and me the news, but after Dr. Ashfaq left she called Sylvia and Monica to tell them.

Sylvia was disconsolate. She knew enough about lung cancer to be very scared for her friend. She knew Lauren would need as much support as possible. In the days ahead she would ask their editor, Ben Weller, if she could take some time off to be with Lauren, to go with her on her doctor appointments; and when she had to go for chemotherapy Sylvia wanted to be able to stay over whenever Lauren needed her to. Monica would request a month, but the editor told her to take all the time off she needed.

In later months, when Lauren's desk was empty, few people besides Lauren's closest friends at *Newsday* knew exactly why. They realized something was not right, but they did not know what. Sylvia later sent out mass e-mails to tell the *Newsday* family what was going on with Lauren.

When Lauren told Monica what Dr. Ashfaq revealed to her about the biopsy, Monica was shocked to hear the confirmation. Lauren admitted that she couldn't believe she was saying it either. Lauren asked Monica if her sister, a nurse at Memorial Sloan-Kettering Cancer Center (MSKCC), could put her in touch with the best surgeon at the hospital. She did, and she recommended a thoracic surgeon, Dr. Raja Flores, who made an appointment to see her just two days later.

Dr. Flores was renowned for his expertise in mesothelioma, lung cancer, and esophageal cancer. Lauren knew she was fortunate to get in to see him that quickly. She learned he was actually squeezing her in between surgeries on that Saturday. He made time in his busy schedule for a consultation with Lauren as well as a man who had come all the way from Italy. From everything Lauren gathered, he was as good as it gets. Three years later, in 2010, he was named chief of thoracic surgery at The Mount Sinai Medical Center and director of the Thoracic Surgical Oncology Program at Mount Sinai Cancer Center.

Sylvia was with her that day. With notebook and pen in hand, she looked every bit the investigative reporter that she was, only now she was not conducting an interview for research on a story, she was just being a good friend; she was taking doctor's notes for her ill and frightened friend.

In his office, Dr. Flores listened intently and sympathetically as Lauren cried through much of the appointment.

Between sobs, Lauren blurted out that that she did not want to die because it would devastate her mother and me. She told him that she was thirty-six and was an only child. He put his hand on her arm and spoke in a calming and reassuring tone. He told her that he was thirty-seven years old and that he was an only child, too. He said that he understood completely, and that he would do everything he could.

Dr. Flores informed her that her cancer was in an advanced stage, 3b, where there were tumors present throughout her chest cavity. He further explained that because there were areas outside her lung that were involved as well, her cancer was technically inoperable. When Sylvia asked what the recommended course of action would be, he said that people whose cancers had spread as far as Lauren's usually receive only chemotherapy and radiation, which tends to shrink the tumors but not always rid the body of them; they are more apt to remain and spread.

Sylvia and Lauren looked at each other. They were thinking the same thing; it all seemed like such a crapshoot.

Dr. Flores saw the distress on their faces and added that he was not ready to let it go at that. He told them if the cancer hadn't metas-tasized to other parts of Lauren's body, such as her brain, he would operate on Lauren even though most doctors faced with a similar case would not attempt it.

Still, this was nothing close to good news. As bad as Lauren's situation appeared when she first walked into Dr. Flores' office, she was still holding out hope that everything would work out for the best. There had still been that possibility less than an hour earlier. Now, as it turned out, the best-case scenario would be Dr. Flores taking out her right lung along with the surrounding tissue in order to remove every trace of the cancer.

The worst case was not something she wanted to think about.

Dr. Flores got up, removed Lauren's films from a file folder, and slapped them against a white light box. He studied them for a moment. "I think I can get this," he said definitively. He made this statement without an ounce of doubt in his voice.

Dr. Flores concluded their consultation by informing Lauren that if she could tolerate the chemotherapy, which he thought she could, that would be his recommended course of treatment, with any follow-up surgery contingent upon how successful the anticancer drugs were in shrinking her tumors.

Sylvia asked when treatment would begin.

"As soon as possible," was his response. He advised Lauren to go home and take as much time as she needed to think about it. "In the meantime, if you have any questions at all, don't hesitate to call me. We'll be ready when you are."

Lauren had such strong confidence in Dr. Flores that she did not want to seek a second opinion from any other surgeon or oncologist.

When Monica called Lauren from Spain later that night and asked how it had gone with Dr. Flores, Lauren told her that she had one of the worst types of cancers, one that was aggressive, returns often, and was in a late stage.

The news landed like an atomic bomb across the Atlantic Ocean. Lauren began crying, but Monica could hardly hear her over her own loud sobs. Monica wished she had not gone on the trip. She wanted to be in New York with Lauren.

Monica asked when her treatment would start and Lauren told her it would begin immediately.

"And if that doesn't work," Lauren added, "I'll need surgery so they can remove my lung."

"How are Frank and Ginny handling it?" Monica asked.

Lauren hesitated before responding. "They still don't know."

"You haven't told them yet?"

"No."

"Oh, Lauren." Monica beseeched Lauren to tell us as soon as possible. "This is way too serious to keep from them this long. They need to know, Lauren. Think how hurt they would be if they found out from someone else."

"I know. I've been wanting to tell them. I just don't know how I'm going to do it." She started to cry again. Through her tears, Lauren said, "I'll go home this weekend. I'll tell them then."

Leah had tried several times to convince Lauren of this very thing. Leah was there when Ginny or I would call. Lauren had been keeping up the pretense that everything was okay when I called. Leah felt terrible hearing Lauren lie to me. She knew this bothered Lauren as well, but Lauren thought she was doing us a favor, protecting us. Leah had previously suggested to Lauren that she come home with her over the weekend to tell us, but it took Monica, who Lauren really looked up to, to convince her to do what she knew was the right thing.

That decision seemed to immediately lighten the load that Lauren had been carrying. Leah could see it on her face. As difficult as the scene would be when she told us what her doctors had discovered, it could only be a tremendous relief to finally put down so much worry during such a difficult time.

Lauren visibly rebounded all at once, and this was amazing for those who witnessed it. She must have been so completely blind-sided by the diagnosis, which all happened so quickly, that it was as if she had just as quickly gotten all her crying and grieving out of the way. Even if it appeared that way, her friends knew Lauren to be a dogged and determined journalist as well as a strong and resilient woman, and they knew these traits had more to do with her courageous outlook than anything else.

After the initial shock wore off, Lauren was not only ready to face the disease but she immediately went to work to figure out how to beat it. Leah knew that Lauren was not the kind of person to take anything lying down. It didn't matter what obstacle she was confronted with, she met it head on. She got herself a thick binder, started taking notes, researched everything she could find about lung cancer, investigated various alternative treatments, and basically looked at all her options. She was willing to try anything, but she was also very practical. She understood the science behind the traditional treatments of chemotherapy and radiation as opposed to nonconventional medicine.

The day after her meeting with Dr. Flores, Lauren had transitioned completely from hysterical to pragmatic, planning for the intense months-long triathlon of chemo, radiation, and surgery that was to follow. She emerged from her previous lethargic state and went somewhere completely unexpected: to Victoria's Secret.

If you were going to get cancer, she reasoned with Sylvia and Leah, you had to have matching bras and panties for those overnight stays at the hospital. Nothing fancy, just black cotton and nylon. She laughed with her friends at the absurdity of trying to buy the right underwear for a potentially terminal illness. Her friends encouraged this indulgence, and Lauren actually felt reasonably sane for the first time in days. It was easy for her to focus on being a normal person when she did something like going out on a shopping spree.

With her underwear crisis resolved, she was ready for chemotherapy. If that went well, she understood that she would be facing surgery to remove a major organ from her body. It seemed inconceivable that she had to come to terms with such a life-altering reality, but she had no other choice.

Lauren did end up seeking the opinions of several other oncologists, all of whom told her pretty much the same thing as Dr. Flores and recommended a similar course of treatment. Lauren also found several diet plans she wanted to try, and talked with her friend Eden about an energy-based healing technique called Reiki, an ancient Japanese practice in which the practitioner's hands, placed on a patient's neural pathways, are believed to generate healing energy.

A subsequent MRI revealed no presence of cancer in Lauren's brain.

She would begin chemotherapy the following week.

4

Lauren had confessed to her friend and coworker Eden that she had been experiencing brief periods when she had difficulty breathing and that she could feel her heart pounding in her chest. Lauren told Eden that she thought her doctor thought she had been suffering from severe anxiety attacks, which could be attributed to her worrying about her mother's medical issue. At the time it made sense to Eden, who had seen firsthand the grave concern Lauren had for her mother's health. Eden and Lauren had gotten to know each on a whole new level after having recently completed the series of assisted-living stories, and Eden could see that Lauren was not well. The reason didn't matter; Eden thought she should have gotten more involved in her friend's well-being.

She wondered how she could have missed all the many signs that pointed to the fact that something was wronged. Like so many others, Eden had been aware of Lauren's puffy, swollen right arm and the purple blood vessel that stood out starkly on the surface of her skin, but cancer never entered her mind. It just did not appear to be that serious. Or she completely dismissed what she was seeing.

It was only after Lauren did not come to work for a couple days that Eden finally snapped out of this catatonia. She tried phoning Lauren several times to find out if she was okay but her calls went unanswered and unreturned. It was Sylvia who urged Lauren to tell Eden about her condition. Sylvia knew Eden was a reporter as well as a friend who would not be ignored. It was quite conceivable that Eden would call us and ask us what was wrong with our daughter.

Having her parents learn about it in such a way was a scenario that Lauren dreaded more than telling us herself.

Eden was stunned when Lauren finally called her back and told her that doctors had found a tumor and that it was lung cancer. When Lauren went on to ask her to be sure not to say anything to us, Eden promised. Like Lauren's other friends, Eden knew how protective Lauren was when it came to her mother and me.

"Why them?" Lauren confided in an e-mail to Eden. "It's not fair that God should take a couple's only child."

Eden understood why Lauren did not immediately tell her about what she was going through. Eden recalled a time when she had initially tested positive for lupus, and at the time she did not even want to so much as say the word out loud because then it would become real. Fortunately, she had gotten a false-positive test result and she was fine. Eden could only hope that her friend and coworker's illness might turn out to be a mistake of some kind as well.

Ten

Lung Cancer: Overlooked, Underfunded

When researchers announced a few weeks ago that rates for breast cancer had dropped a staggering 7 percent between 2002 and 2003, the news was hailed by an advocacy movement that has fought tirelessly in the past few decades to raise awareness and money for a cure.

The decline in large part was attributed to women drastically abandoning hormone replacement therapy after a myriad of studies suggested a link between estrogen and breast cancer.

If only the strides were as promising with lung cancer and some of the other cancers that have failed to get as much attention, media ink and research dollars through the years.

I believe in truth in advertising, so I must disclose I am one of the hundreds of thousands of women in America battling lung cancer. Let's face it: Though it's the biggest cancer killer among men and women, lung cancer remains the Ugly Betty of cancers, the one few want to acknowledge, the one that has a barely recognizable ribbon. It's a sickly-looking, unattractive clear ribbon—because lung cancer has often been perceived by advocates as the "invisible" disease—as opposed to the ubiquitous bright pink ribbon that has become the emblem of the breast cancer movement. This is not to say that breast cancer doesn't deserve the attention it has received. It does, since one in eight women will get it in their lifetimes.

But lung cancer is the cancer that is still whispered in elevators or crowded rooms. It is the cancer that immediately elicits the question, "How long did you smoke?" In the end, it doesn't really matter.

Blame is a wasted effort, and we're all in this together, aren't we? As a society, we should be vigorously seeking all potential cures for all cancers. I hope so.

But in my travels in cancer land during the past few years, I've disappointingly found that a caste system of cancers does exist, at least when it comes to funding and public awareness.

—From *Newsday*, "Life, with Cancer," January 9, 2007, "Lung Cancer: Overlooked, Underfunded," by Lauren Terrazzano

1

There are two major types of lung cancer, small cell lung cancer (SCLC) and non-small cell lung cancer (NSCLC). The two are distinguished histologically as well by how they are treated, with non-small cell lung cancer being primarily treated with surgery, if feasible, while small cell lung carcinoma is more frequently treated with chemotherapy and radiation. If the lung cancer has characteristics of both types it is called a mixed small cell/large cell carcinoma, which is very uncommon.

About 85 to 90 percent of lung cancers are of the NSCLC variety, with three main subtypes: squamous cell (epidermoid) carcinoma; adenocarcinoma; and large cell (undifferentiated) carcinoma. The cells in each of these subtypes differ in size, shape, and chemical makeup, but are grouped together because the approach to treatment and prognosis are very similar. In breaking down these subtypes of NSCLC, about 25 to 30 percent of all lung cancers are squamous cell (epidermoid) carcinomas. These cancers start in early versions of squamous cells, which are flat cells that line the inside of the airways in the lungs. They are often linked to a history of smoking and tend to be found in the middle of the lungs, near a bronchus. About 40 percent of lung cancers are adenocarcinomas. These cancers start in early versions of the cells that would normally secrete substances such as mucus. This type of lung cancer occurs mainly in people who smoke or have smoked, but it is also the most common type of lung cancer seen in nonsmokers. It is more common in women than in men, and it is more likely to occur in younger people than other types of lung cancer. Adenocarcinoma is usually found in the outer region of the lung. It tends to grow more slowly than other types of lung cancer and is more likely to be found before it has spread outside of the lung. Large cell (undifferentiated) carcinoma is a third main type of non-small cell lung cancer, and accounts for about 10 to 15 percent of lung cancers. It may appear in any part of the lung. It tends to grow and spread quickly, which can make it harder to treat. A subtype of large cell carcinoma known as large cell neuroendocrine carcinoma is a fast-growing cancer that is very similar to small cell lung cancer.

Considering small cell lung cancer (SCLC), which accounts for about 10 to 15 percent of all lung cancers, this second major type of lung cancer is named for the small cells that make up these cancers. Small cell lung cancer occurs almost exclusively in smokers, particularly heavy smokers, and tends to grow and spread quickly and widely through the body fairly early in the course of the disease, usually before symptoms are detected. Because of this, surgery is considered a positive step less often in patients with small cell lung cancer than with non-small cell lung cancer. Chemotherapy is an important part of treatment for all small cell lung cancers, as long as a person is healthy enough to tolerate it.

Cancers that start in other organs, such as the breast, pancreas, kidney, or skin can sometimes spread, or metastasize, to the lungs, but these are not lung cancers. A cancer that starts in the breast and spreads to the lungs is still breast cancer, not lung cancer. Treatment for metastatic cancer to the lungs depends on where it started.

Lauren had small cell lung cancer. For the purpose of treatment, a person with small cell lung cancer is classified as having either limited disease or extensive disease.

In people with limited lung disease, the cancer is present within the lung on only one side of the chest and/or in the central lymph nodes. About one-third of patients with small cell lung cancer have limited disease at the time they are diagnosed. However, in almost all cases, the cancer will have spread outside of the chest in a way that is not yet visible with imaging tests. Most people with limited disease are treated with chemotherapy in combination with radiation therapy. In early stages, one or two, surgery should be considered, although these cases are rare.

In patients with extensive lung disease, the cancer has spread to the other side of the chest or to more distant locations in the body. Patients are generally given chemotherapy as the initial treatment; surgery is not an option. People who respond to chemotherapy are often given radiation therapy to the brain to prevent the development of brain metastases.

Lauren displayed many of the disease's clinical features, including chest pain, weight loss, malaise, and distension of the superficial veins of the head and neck. In Lauren's case, these symptoms were discovered too late, however, so surgery to remove the lung tumor was not even considered since it would not improve the probability (or length) of her survival.

Only in a small number of these cases would surgery be beneficial—less than 10 percent—and only among those who had been diagnosed very early in the course of their disease. In these patients, surgery followed by chemotherapy can result in a five-year survival rate of up to 35 to 40 percent.

Chemotherapy is of clear benefit in patients with small cell lung cancer and is a mainstay treatment. Chemotherapy works by interfering with the ability of rapidly growing cells such as cancer cells to divide or reproduce themselves. Because most of an adult's normal cells are not actively growing, they are not affected as much by chemotherapy, with the exception of bone marrow, where the blood cells are produced, the hair, and the lining of the gastrointestinal tract. However, normal cells as well as cancer cells are affected by these chemicals, giving rise to a wide range of side effects.

Due to the effect of chemotherapy on bone marrow, the most important side effect of chemotherapy is a corresponding and transient drop in the blood counts, which can increase the chances of developing life-threatening infections, such as pneumonia. During treatment, patients are closely monitored for these side effects and any signs of toxicity, which typically occur one to two weeks after chemotherapy begins. Other possible side effects of chemotherapy include fatigue, hair loss, nausea, numbness in the fingers and toes, hearing loss, diarrhea, and changes in kidney function.

A number of chemotherapy drugs are presently being used against small cell lung cancer, with many new drugs continually being explored. A single chemotherapy drug may be used to treat small cell lung cancer, although combination therapy is more common, with two or more drugs given together. This improves the chance of reducing the size of the tumor, referred to as a response to therapy, and modestly lengthens survival. Chemotherapy is usually administered intravenously, although some agents can be given by mouth.

Generally speaking, chemotherapy is administered over a one- to three-day period, usually every three weeks, and then repeated. The short period of drug administration followed by the waiting period is called one cycle of chemotherapy. Four to six cycles are typically recommended.

Radiation therapy (RT) is often recommended during chemotherapy for people with limited small-cell lung cancer. Radiation therapy involves the use of focused, high energy X–rays to destroy cancer cells. The x-rays are delivered from a machine called a linear accelerator. Individual treatments are brief, typically ten to fifteen minutes, and not painful.

The damaging effect of radiation is cumulative, and a certain amount of radiation must be delivered before the cancer cells are so damaged that they die. To accomplish this, small radiation doses are administered daily, five days per week, for five to seven weeks. Radiation is only administered to the areas of the body that are affected by the tumor. In contrast to chemotherapy, which is a systemic treatment, radiation is a local treatment, and side effects are generally limited to the area undergoing radiation.

The best way of combining chest radiation therapy with chemotherapy is a debatable issue, although most experts believe that the benefit of each treatment is greater when they are given concurrently and begun at the same time. The side effects of both treatments are usually more pronounced, including lowering of the blood counts, difficulty swallowing due to inflammation of the lining of the esophagus, and inflammation of the normal lung surrounding the tumor. Chest RT can sometimes be given after chemotherapy has been completed; this is called sequential therapy.

The side effects of radiation occur gradually over the weeks of treatment. They include fatigue, possible mild reddening of skin, and esophageal symptoms characterized by an initial feeling of a "lump in one's throat" when swallowing, and eventually a sore throat. The esophageal symptoms are closely monitored and treated with appropriate pain medications. Long-term side effects occur many months after radiation has been completed and include scarring of the unaffected lung and sometimes shortness of breath.

The brain is a common site of metastasis in people with small cell lung cancer. Having preventive radiation treatment of the brain after chemotherapy, before evidence of metastases develops, can substantially reduce the chances of developing brain metastases and prolong survival.

Small cell lung cancer is more responsive to chemotherapy and radiation therapy than other cell types of lung cancer, though a cure remains difficult to achieve because SCLC has a greater tendency to be widely disseminated by the time of diagnosis. This was the case with Lauren when her cancer was discovered. Without any chemotherapy, the average survival is measured in weeks. The likelihood of responding to chemotherapy, with or without radiation therapy, is quite high. Response rates of 80 to 100 percent are seen in patients with limited disease, when the cancer is diagnosed early enough, and approximately one-half of these are complete.

With extensive stage disease, and late detection, 60 to 80 percent of patients will respond to chemotherapy, and between 15 and 40 percent will have a complete response.

Despite these favorable results, small cell lung cancer tends to recur or relapse within one to two years in the majority of patients, particularly those with extensive stage disease. If the small cell lung cancer recurs or fails to respond to one type of chemotherapy regimen, a different type of chemotherapy regimen may offer some relief from symptoms and a modest improvement in the chances of survival.

Regardless of stage, however, and despite improvements in diagnosis and therapy made in recent years, the current prognosis for patients with SCLC is not very good. Without treatment, SCLC has the most aggressive clinical course of any type of pulmonary tumor, with median survival from diagnosis of only two to four months. About 10 percent of the total population of SCLC patients remains free of disease during the two years from the start of therapy, which is the time period during which most relapses occur. Even these patients, however, are at risk of dying from lung cancer. The overall survival at five years is 5 to 10 percent.

Lauren knew all this, and looking it up, she knew she was part of these statistics.

2

After nine days in Spain, Monica returned home just as Lauren was about to begin her first round of chemotherapy. She was with Lauren when she walked into Sloan-Kettering for the first time.

This was where Lauren had been scheduled to begin the first of three rounds of chemotherapy, with the goal of shrinking her tumors. Not only is this facility the oldest and largest private cancer center in the world, it had been considered one of the nation's premier cancer centers since its founding in 1884. Lauren was aware of the hospital's reputation as an exceptional patient care and leading-edge research facility and she had confided to her friends that she felt quite confident knowing that she would not be fighting her cancer alone. Taking a stand against the disease and defending her body would be the very latest technology and medicines, along with a team of talented and devoted surgeons who performed more cancer operations than at any other hospital. She would never have gone so far as to say she had a distinct advantage over the disease, but she liked her chances.

Still, walking into a facility that was a veritable war zone in a mortal battle between humanity and all manner of cancers was frightening for Lauren. These were the frontlines. People came here to have cancer cells destroyed and tumors shrunk. Paradoxically, the atmosphere was more than pleasant. In fact, if patients somehow didn't know what they were really doing there, they might have thought they were treating themselves to a visit at some upscale Manhattan spa for a day of pampering.

The entrance to Sloan-Kettering's Outpatient Cancer Center was not canopied and red-carpeted, but once you were inside on the upper floors of the chemotherapy treatment suites, you were afforded just about every other convenience available.

Lauren immediately noticed the benches that lined the interior of the elevators. The tan upholstered seats perplexed her at first. She wondered for a moment just how far up they were going. Images of the final sequence in *Willy Wonka & the Chocolate Factory* came to mind, when they burst through the factory roof in the Wonkavator, a multidirectional glass elevator. Lauren knew she was in for an adventure of her own, and she didn't know where it would take her, but this was where it was beginning.

Lauren stepped out of the elevator and entered a room with leather couches and walls of trickling water. The soft, melodic music being piped in added to the soothing setting, but it could not quite calm Lauren down. The packets of tea and graham crackers in the corner could not, either. But the televisions, all showing *Live with Regis and Kelly*, brought everything crashing back to reality for her. The hosts laughing and joking, having such a blissful time without a worry in the world, perhaps was intended to take the cancer patient's mind off their worries for a moment or two, but for Lauren the trite and mundane banter only underscored the absurdity of where she was and what she was facing. This was hell's waiting room, Lauren thought.

This moment of epiphany was one of several Lauren would experience in the near future, a future she was suddenly unsure about. She wanted to remain positive, but it was not easy. As she looked around and observed some of her fellow cancer suffers, it was impossible not to notice that most of them were decades older than she was. Because lung cancer can take years to develop, it is mostly found in older people, with seventy-one being the average age that a person receives a lung cancer diagnosis. So Lauren could not help feeling disconnected from them as well as from her condition. Every time she looked at it, it was the same thing: she was just thirty-six years old. She should have been contemplating her future, not her funeral, but she was diagnosed with a disease that she knew was frequently a death sentence.

She knew she did not fit the classic profile of a lung cancer patient, at least the old stereotype of a sixty-year-old man who has smoked all of his life. Hers was the lung cancer for a new generation, and Lauren was afraid she had unwittingly become its poster child.

Lung cancer, as it turns out, is quite far-reaching in this day and age. As one of the most common cancers, it is certainly no secret. However, its true impact on the human population cannot be fully grasped without citing some numbing statistics. Lauren did not want to diminish the personal suffering that any cancer patient (and his or her family) experienced, but she thought it was useful to separate the individual from the disease, if only to highlight the staggering numbers involved. Lauren, too, was more than just a statistic, but she was shocked by some of the raw data that was readily available for all to see. When she came across them herself, she felt compelled to share this knowledge with others, at the very least her family and friends.

In recent years, lung cancer has comprised approximately 15 percent of all cancer diagnoses and 30 percent of all cancer deaths. Lung cancer surpassed breast cancer as the number one cancer killer of women in 1987. It kills nearly twice as many women as breast cancer and nearly three times as many men as prostate cancer. In fact, lung cancer kills more people than breast, prostate, colon, liver, kidney, and melanoma cancers *combined*. It claims nearly 450 American lives every day, 160,000 per year. Every three minutes someone in the United States is diagnosed with lung cancer. It is the second most diagnosed cancer in men and women, after prostate cancer and breast cancer, respectively.

Cigarette smoking is still the primary cause of most lung cancers, but there are other factors that must also be considered. Every year in the United States, lung cancers in people who have never smoked kill more people than AIDS. Sometimes, a person develops lung cancer and doctors do not know why. Secondhand smoke is believed to be the number-two contributing factor in the prevalence of lung cancer.

Beyond being responsible for tens of thousands of deaths every year, including about 3,400 lung cancer deaths and an estimated 46,000 heart disease deaths, secondhand smoke might also play a role in the development of breast cancer. Furthermore, children exposed to secondhand smoke not only suffer respiratory diseases, asthma attacks, and infections at higher rates than those who are not exposed, experts believe it is a direct link to a host of other children's health issues—a list that includes pneumonia, bronchitis, and even SIDS. Secondhand smoke has also been shown to harm fetuses. Pregnant women exposed to secondhand smoke have more miscarriages and stillbirths, an increased risk of delivering a baby with low birth weight, and more babies with impaired lung function.

In the search for other causes for the prevalence of lung cancer among nonsmokers, Lauren found studies by the American Lung Association that indicated that particle pollution kills an estimated 13,000 people per year. The poor are often exposed to the highest levels of pollutants because lower income frequently means living in close proximity to power plants and highways and in heavily polluted inner cities. A recent State of the Air quality report by the American

Lung Association noted that more than 154 million people—half the country's population—are threatened by dangerously high pollution levels.

Some research has indicated that food additives may be responsible for the increase and spread of lung cancer. Gene studies are being conducted to see what ties heredity and nationality have to the incidence of lung cancer. Other studies have been able to link certain occupations with an increased risk of developing lung cancer, such as truck drivers regularly exposed to diesel exhaust.

Lung cancer and pancreatic cancer are among the most difficult to detect early, but scanning methods to quickly identify cancer in the blood are in development. Drug trials are also underway that may prove effective against particular types of cancers, including lung cancer.

While the connection between smoking and cancer is no longer doubted, Lauren was among the 15 percent of women with lung cancer who were considered nonsmokers, even though she did smoke infrequently for a short period of time. And while I smoked until 1990, I rarely did so around Lauren when she was a child. She never blamed me, but she confided to me later that not a day went by since that August afternoon in 2004 that she did not wonder if she might have been spared if she had never picked up a cigarette.

Lung cancer is largely perceived as a self-inflicted disease, and no one could tell Lauren whether her occasional smoking caused her cancer; but in her darkest moments she blamed herself. She knew there were plenty of others who did as well, as she quickly found out. Society tends to pillory people for illnesses that can be caused by bad habits. Such a stigma cast upon lung cancer patients is always unfair, but particularly so for people who never smoked a day in their lives.

3

In her research, Lauren learned that lung cancer was in many ways a woman's disease. At the start of the twenty-first century, lung cancer killed more than 70,000 women each year in the United States alone, a mortality that is greater than the number of women's lives claimed each year by breast, ovarian, and uterine cancers combined. In addition, women younger than forty have been found to have a slightly greater risk of developing the disease than men under that age, a fact Lauren had discovered from the American Cancer Society in Atlanta. Rates of the disease in men have leveled over the previous quarter century, while rates among women have increased. According to a study in the *Journal of the American Medical Association* published at that time, Lauren discovered that women who smoke were shown to be almost twice as likely to get lung cancer as male smokers.

Lauren continued to learn more as she went further and further along in her treatment. For a reporter, the facts were relatively easy to come by, though as a sufferer, she found them very difficult to face and to digest. Lauren understood why anyone would just want to shut their eyes to the harsher truths about lung cancer, but she could not. There was so much that was unknown about the disease. So much that was unclear, shrouded by myth and misconceptions. And of what was understood about lung cancer, few people seemed to know, much less care. She wanted to bring all of these things out in the open, to reach as many people as she could.

The little attention that was paid specifically to the incidence of the disease in women in both public perception and medical research funding was an aspect of lung cancer that Lauren saw as an affront, and she hoped she could help change the perception among some women that it could not happen to them even if they did not smoke. While the statistics were frightening, Lauren joked with friends that there were no cute pink ribbons, not even any tar-brown ribbons, for lung cancer, few nationwide walks for a cure, and no celebrity spokespersons who had had the disease. While there have certainly been a good number of celebrities who have fallen victim to lung cancer, Lauren was always quick to point out that they usually don't live long enough to advocate for awareness and research dollars. Some stars who died due to lung cancer include Bing Crosby, Dean Martin, Paul Newman, George Harrison, John Wayne, and Walt Disney. This short list noticeably consists only of men, all of a past era (except for Harrison, who died in 2001), and many were heavy smokers. But there have been well-known women, as well, who have succumbed to lung cancer, among them Rosemary Clooney, Betty Grable, Susan Hayward, and Amanda Blake ("Miss Kitty" from Gunsmoke); and some reports have mentioned smoking-induced lung cancer as a contributing factor in the death of Lucille Ball, though the official cause was listed as heart disease. These women were from another era, like most of the men, and presumably smoked. It was not until Dana Reeve, the courageous wife of actor Christopher Reeve, developed lung cancer as a nonsmoker and died of the disease in 2006 that the public got its first real inkling of what this disease was really all about. Dana Reeve's death should have been a wake-up call for women, but Lauren would say that too many young girls (in particular) just hit the snooze alarm instead.

Lung cancer in women differs from lung cancer in men in many fundamental ways, including the causes, response to various treatments, survival rate, and even the symptoms. Overall, lung cancer still affects men more than women, but the gap is closing. Additionally, lung cancer in women has also been found to occur at a slightly younger age, with women under the age of fifty being particularly vulnerable. The reason for this is also not fully understood, although there have been several studies that suggest women are more susceptible to the carcinogens in cigarettes, and thus tend to develop lung cancer after fewer years of smoking.

Even though smoking remains the number-one cause of lung cancer in women, just as it is for men, recent studies indicate that women who smoke may actually be more likely to develop lung cancer than men who smoke. While some of the other recognized causes of lung cancer—secondhand smoke, exposure to radon in homes, various noxious environmental and occupational exposures, and genetic predispositions—are the same for both sexes, recent studies suggest infection with the human papillomavirus may also play a role in female susceptibility to the disease. Human papillomavirus, more commonly known as HPV, is a viral infection spread through skin-to-skin sexual contact and has been linked in the past with increased incidences of cervical cancer.

It is likely that estrogen also plays a role in the development and progression of lung cancer, and research is currently being done to define this further. Women who have their ovaries removed surgically before menopause may be at higher risk of developing lung cancer. Recent research suggests that treatment with estrogen and progesterone (hormone replacement therapy) after menopause may increase the risk of dying from lung cancer, though it did not increase the risk of developing lung cancer.

With regard to cancer type, whereas men are more likely to develop squamous cell lung cancer, another form of non-small cell lung cancer, adenocarcinoma is the most common type of lung cancer found in women. BAC (bronchioalveolar carcinoma) is a rare form of lung cancer that is more common in women. For unknown reasons, the incidence of BAC appears to be increasing worldwide, especially among younger, nonsmoking women.

Much has been made about the symptoms of a heart attack being different in women than in men, and the same appears to hold true for lung cancer. The most common type of lung cancer found in men often presents itself with the "classic" symptoms—an obvious and persistent cough, or even coughing up blood. The type of lung cancer that is more common in women can grow quite large and spread before any symptoms appear. Often, the onset of fatigue, gradual shortness of breath, or chest and back pain due to the spread of lung cancer to the bones come too late as the first signs that something is wrong.

Historically, women have responded to a few lung cancer chemotherapy medications better than their male counterparts. And women who are able to be treated with surgery for lung cancer also tend to fare better. In one study, the median survival after surgery for lung cancer was twice as long for women as for men. On the other hand, even though the National Cancer Institute recommends that all patients with stage three lung cancer be considered candidates for clinical trials, women are less likely to be involved in clinical trials than men.

The rate of survival for women with lung cancer is only slightly higher than it is for men at all stages of the disease, with a 16 percent overall five-year survival rate compared to 12 percent for men.

Increased awareness and funding for research is something lung cancer advocates continue to push for. It is by no means a popularity contest or a competition, for which the disease with the highest mortality rate wins the prize money. It's about recognition and preserving life. There are a great many obstacles that must be overcome: the low survival rate and the challenge of early detection, not to mention the stigma associated with smoking.

Prevention still remains the best medicine, but even avoiding cigarette smoke and radon does not keep a person safe from lung cancer. There remains no cure, and the best a woman with lung cancer can hope for is a 16 percent chance of survival, with a five-year survival rate.

Eleven

Focusing on
Present Matters the Most

"*Two to three months,*" *the doctor said, almost reluctantly, when I finally posed the question. That's eight to twelve weeks. Sixty to 90 days. Or 2,160 hours, if you want to get right down to it.*

I don't know what possessed me to ask the oncologist how long I have left. In the nearly three years I've been battling this disease, I've never asked for my prognosis. I hate that word. But my body has betrayed me lately, more than usual. I've had a rough couple of weeks, with news of my cancer spreading, new blood clots, and fluid buildup in my abdomen, which has made it difficult to breathe.

There seem to be no more weapons left in the arsenal. Chemo is no longer an option; nothing seems to work. I've had so much surgery I feel like the Bionic Woman: "We can rebuild her." But with each operation, it has been harder and harder, quite frankly, to rebuild me.

Whether the oncologist is right, no one knows. These white-coated mortals do their best and make their best guesses based on data and statistics and other cases. But death, like life, is not a precise science. Only fate knows. What I know for certain is that I am 39. I have seen people like my grandfather live simple but happy long lives. He died when he was 93. On the opposite end, in my job as a reporter, I have seen 3-year-olds die at the hands of abusive parents. Nothing really makes sense when it comes to death.

Still, I was hoping you wouldn't notice the recent absence of my column; I was wrong. Apparently there are more readers out there than my parents and my husband. I didn't want to tackle this subject in this space. I had more cerebral, complicated topics in mind. Like the most recent controversial study surrounding the benefits of early CT scan screening for lung cancer, or the recent, sickening push by one tobacco company to market its traditionally male-oriented brand of cigarette to young women. I hope to eventually get to those topics.

—From *Newsday,* "Life, with Cancer," April 10, 2007, "Focusing on Present Matters the Most," by Lauren Terrazzano

1

After the first round of chemo at Memorial Sloan-Kettering Cancer Center, Lauren was no longer able to work. She tried, but she was just too sick. It was hard for her to eat, and she became weaker by the day. Nothing tasted right. She even lost her love of chocolate. What little food she ate she had trouble keeping down.

Lauren received her second round of chemotherapy at Massachusetts General Hospital in Boston, so she was able to stay with us during that time. However, complications from the side effects of the anticancer drugs landed Lauren in intensive care on separate occasions when she developed two very tenacious, life-threatening infections. It was a harrowing time for her mother and for me as we watched our daughter clinging to life on the brink of death before she finally managed to pull out of it and regain enough strength to fight off the infection.

While she was recovering from the second episode in Mass General, her friends Tomoeh and Archie took it upon themselves to arrive the day before and clean the place from top to bottom. That was much more than a lovely gesture made by dear friends. Because of Lauren's suppressed immune system, it was important for her health that she come home to an apartment that was immaculate and as sterile as an apartment in New York can be. Tomoeh also took the time to decorate the place with brightly colored origami figures that she had made. Crafting the animals and shapes out of paper was something she had learned as a child growing up in Japan. Tomoeh also bought Lauren a binder so she could organize all of her doctors' notes, lab tests, and other information. She even took a day off work to help Lauren arrange everything. From that moment on, Lauren always had that notebook with her—not unlike her copies of Nancy Drew mysteries that she toted around everywhere she went as a teen.

By the third round of chemo, back in New York at Sloan-Kettering, Lauren had become one of those people who had to sit down on the benches in the Wonkavator for the ride up to the chemotherapy suites. She experienced another setback early on at the start of the cycle when she developed a blood clot in her left leg and then for rest of the treatment had to give herself a daily injection of blood thinners. Throughout all this, Lauren had no idea if the tumors in her chest were growing or shrinking, or whether or not what she was putting her body through was worth it.

By the end, she felt physically awful and emotionally devastated. She did not want to go anywhere or be seen by anyone. Her long, straight chestnut hair had been falling out, first in strands, then in massive clumps that would come out in the shower. She used to love twirling her hair around her finger when she was bored.

One day, in a fit of anger, she grabbed a pair of scissors and lopped off what was left of her locks. She then quietly arranged for her hairstylist to come to her apartment to try to salvage what was left, but she hadn't left much to work with. Lauren could not embrace the female equivalent of the comb-over, so she went out and got a wig. She hated it from the very beginning; it was uncomfortable, hot, and itchy. Her friends did everything they could to boost her spirits, buying her a variety of hats in different styles and colors. Someone even bought her giant orange earrings.

"You think these gaudy things are going to somehow disguise the fact I'm bald," Lauren joked. "If they were a little bigger they would cover my head completely."

Mostly, Lauren wore a soft blue cotton cap to warm her cold head or just a simple Boston Red Sox cap.

Unable to maintain her weight, she got skinnier by the day. Lauren found it brutally ironic that shedding weight with such ease, something she had dreamed about during healthier days, now terrified her.

It was also a time when Lauren found out who in her life was a real friend—who was there for her when she needed them most. Coworkers and colleagues came to see her, friends visited and tried to keep her entertained, including bringing her back issues of *People*, among other tabloid publications.

Whenever they could, Lauren's friends would take her out into the cold, harsh light of day for a walk in the park. Her mother and I came down from Boston during the week to take care of her.

2

When the doctors gathered to determine the results of Lauren's treatment, they reported to her that the tumors had not shrunk. The cancer cells certainly were less active and had not grown, but they did not shrink. This was not a promising sign. With no improvement, surgery could not reasonably be recommended. An operation at that point was considered too dangerous and would not have been helpful to Lauren in any way. Instead, a fourth cycle of chemotherapy was suggested, and Lauren grudgingly consented.

The result, however, was the same: no improvement.

Lauren's doctors were stymied as to how to treat Lauren's cancer at that point. They told her that any further chemotherapy was futile. These powerful anticancer drugs were not getting the job done, and surgery would do nothing to stop the proliferation of the cancer cells. They felt they had run out of options. I could not accept that, and to his credit, neither could Dr. Flores. He went before the hospital's tumor board and made a case to get Lauren into the operating room and give him a chance to see if he could do something more for her. Although the board voted against the risky surgery, Dr. Flores managed to convince them that removing the infected lung would be the only thing that would save her life, and finally they acquiesced. When he consulted with Lauren, Dr. Flores told her that an aggressive approach was necessary, and she agreed.

Dr. Flores was cautiously optimistic. He told Lauren, "I think we can get this thing." In December, Dr. Flores thought Lauren was strong enough for the surgery, and the procedure was scheduled for later that month. All Lauren could do was prepare herself, particularly mentally, as best she could. She knew that the surgery would be long and complicated, and that she might die. Any surgery is fraught with risks, such as cardiac arrest or bleeding to death. The removal of a major organ, like a lung, only increased the danger. Nothing was guaranteed.

Despite the possible dire consequences, Lauren remained hopeful. Most of all, she trusted Dr. Flores, though prior to the operation she did take the precaution of having her will drawn up. She said her good-byes to her closest friends and to us, just in case she did not survive.

The night before going to the hospital she prayed, something she had been doing a lot of lately. She did not know what to expect. She found it surreal to think that she was going to have a major organ removed from her body, and she was scared. The following morning, December 17, she went under the knife.

3

Dr. Flores performed what is known as an extrapleural pneumo-nectomy on Lauren, taking out her right lung along with its lining, part of her diaphragm, and the outer lining of her heart. He removed all the cancer that he could see, and the surgery was considered a success.

We felt Lauren seemed to recover remarkably well, considering everything. She was smiling and joking from the moment she got out of surgery, and within a couple of days she was happy to be celebrating Christmas with us and with her friends. She finally appeared to be turning the corner, but her resurgence was short-lived: just three weeks later she started a six-week course of radiation therapy.

The technicians "tattooed" her chest, precisely marking the location where they were going to guide the beam. This was a time when Lauren was most sick, throwing up practically every day. The treatments really knocked her for a loop. When she wasn't on her knees in the bathroom, she would flop onto the bed when she got home from a session and usually would not emerge from her room until the next day—just in time for another dose of radiation. To make matters worse, Lauren disliked her radiologist, who was insensitive and rude to her even as she was fighting for her life.

She lost all the weight, and then some, that she had managed to put back on over the holidays following her surgery. Her appearance was ghostly. She was in so much pain that she could barely walk, and there were times when she did not think she was going to make it through another day. It was pure torture for her mother and me to witness this.

After Lauren completed her treatment, in early March she started to feel a little better and tests showed that she was, indeed, cancer-free. Having endured so much, it suddenly appeared that it had all been worth it. For the first time since she had been diagnosed with lung cancer, Lauren truly felt good for an extended period of time. Her hair started to grow back, only instead of coming back in straight, it came back curly. Her strength also returned, and she slowly started to put on weight.

Lauren's idea of real progress came the month after her treatment ended. She had taken a trip to Florida and she'd eaten pizza, her first bite of solid food in months. It tasted as good as the finest gourmet meal she'd ever had. She spent the rest of the vacation relaxing on the beach, soaking up vitamin D from the sun, and floating in the crystal-clear waters of Florida and just feeling alive.

By May she was preparing to get back to work, at least part-time. Everyone at *Newsday* was happy to have her back, and she was overjoyed to return. However, she had a difficult time at first, writing stories about other people's tragedies and triumphs. Lauren's ambivalence about her future had her emotions going in several directions at once. There were times she became angry; at other times, she couldn't stop crying. If she was working on a story about someone who was facing cancer or some other life-threatening disease, she would be profoundly affected. As a professional, she got the job done, but her friends at *Newsday* saw how much it bothered her.

This is not something her mother or I were aware of at that time. Even at that stage, Lauren continued to try to shield us from as much bad news as possible.

Tomoeh had gone with Lauren to see her oncologist on several occasions. In between the visits, Lauren seemed to be fine, but in the days leading up to an appointment she would be filled with such dread that her friend could hear a tremble in her voice when she spoke. Sometimes she would cry when there was a message on her answering machine from her doctors and she had to call them back. These calls, or any unusual pain or feeling in her body that she was not familiar with, would trigger a panic attack and she would think that the cancer had returned.

Once Tomoeh was in the car with Lauren when she began crying after her cell phone rang and she saw that her doctor was calling her. Lauren had to pull the car over until Lauren calmed down. When she was composed enough to return the call to the doctor, she found out that it was nothing, just a scheduling issue. This time.

Lauren continued checking in with the doctor to make sure the cancer had not returned. The anxiety, though, never really dissipated; it was just something Lauren had to deal with. There was simply no choice in the matter. Her anxiety was pervasive and upset Ginny and me as well as Lauren's friends; we had to find our own way of coping with it. Lauren saw how her attitude and temperament affected us, and she was deeply concerned. At one point Lauren suggested that all her friends go to see a therapist to make sure they were okay. She was particularly worried about her mother and me, and she asked her friends to watch out for us.

Then Lauren learned that Amy, her friend in treatment at Sloan-Kettering, had had a recurrence and was undergoing further chemotherapy. During late-night phone conversations, the two women would avoid the temptation of pitying themselves, but they did talk about their rage and their fears, the kind that crept up on them and made them want to punch their fists through a wall—or else hide under the covers in the morning. Talking with Amy helped Lauren make a resolution to move on, to live life between the CT scans every three months to the fullest, and to try not to go out of her mind with worry that something was going to show up on the scan.

When Amy got sick again, Lauren figured that she owed it to herself, and everyone else, not to let her medical condition keep her down. She was determined to spend more time traveling, being with us and her friends, and just enjoying her life with all the people she was fortunate enough to share it with. Her newfound health enabled her to go on excursions to places like the Bahamas and Iceland, and she savored every moment of her freedom from the chemotherapy infusion center at Sloan-Kettering.

On the outside, Lauren was starting to look like her old self, even though her hair had grown back with dark curls. But getting her hair cut was not an option—she didn't care how much her friends taunted her with shouts of, "Hey, broccoli head." Maybe it was vanity, but after losing her hair to cancer, she didn't want to lose it again, even to a hairdresser's scissors. She also went out and bought an exorbitant amount of lip gloss, something she had not been particularly big on in the past. She came to terms with the large L-shaped scar extending down her chest and under her right breast. When she was in a department store's dressing room trying on new clothes, she would simply turn her back on the full-length mirror while she slipped into the outfit and then turn back around to see how she looked. And each time she returned to Sloan-Kettering for a doctor's appointments, she was grateful to be standing, not sitting, in the elevator.

4

In September, Lauren organized a charity hike up Bear Mountain, one of the best-known peaks of New York's Hudson Highlands and located within the 5,000-acre Bear Mountain State Park, about forty miles north of Manhattan. Its 1,300-foot summit is accessible by a paved road and crisscrossed by several hiking trails, including the oldest section of the Appalachian Trail. At the top is an observation tower that offers magnificent views of Bear Mountain Bridge and the Hudson River. To the south, the skyline of Manhattan is visible on clear days. The mountain was given the name by early explorers who thought its varied peaks resembled a sleeping bear.

Lauren led friends, colleagues, and their families up the mountain to raise money for lung cancer research. Collin Nash of *Newsday* was among the hikers happy to be there for Lauren and to support the cause she was sponsoring. They had both been at the paper for some time, but it wasn't until they began sitting next to each other that they began to develop a friendship. He began to call her "Baby Girl," a term of endearment that he used for both his wife and his teenage daughter. Prior to that, from afar, Collin had always admired Lauren for her tireless work ethic and unrelenting passion for her craft.

Lauren was such a go-getter, Collin often joked with her, telling her she needed to relax a little, that she needed to have more balance in her life and not let her life revolve solely around her career. When she started to complain about being tired all the time, Collin chided her for not paying more attention to her health. In fact, at his urging she had begun a workout regimen after she'd expressed concern to him about the swollen welts that had appeared on her arm.

Collin had been impressed with the courage Lauren displayed while fighting tooth and nail for her life for the past year. She somehow managed to remain positive even after a number of major setbacks. In fact, it was his understanding that Lauren came up with the idea to celebrate the completion of her treatment and her future recovery by climbing Bear Mountain after a particularly grueling fourth cycle of chemotherapy. She started planning for the event even before she had gotten word that the cancer had been halted.

Lauren did not expect so many willing participants. She thought it would be just herself and a couple of her friends, but more than forty people showed up. With her energy level still rebounding from the exhaustive treatment regimen she had endured, she was determined to claw her way up the mountain, and she did so with relative ease, making the four-mile climb to the peak in ninety minutes.

Lauren was so elated by her accomplishment, and so grateful to all those who joined her, that she gave her fellow climbers commemorative T-shirts as her way of thanking them. The front of the Dr. Seuss-themed shirts read: "So . . . be your name Buxman or Bixby or Bray or Mordecai Ali Van Allen O'Shea. Today is your day! Your mountain is waiting. So . . . get on your way!"

5

Lauren lived cancer-free for the next six months, the culmination of which was an unexpected wedding.

Right after Lauren got sick, Al came back into the picture. At this time, I had no problems with him. Ginny's opinion of him hadn't changed. She made it clear to me that she didn't care for him, but I gave him the benefit of the doubt. That's just how I am. An eternal optimist, perhaps, or just a fool, but I actually defended him. Ginny and I got into arguments over it.

Then Lauren called late one night from Lake George, New York, a resort where she and Al were vacationing over the Labor Day weekend in 2005. Excitedly, Lauren told us that Al had proposed and that they had decided to get married in the spring. Ginny and I were both very happy to hear this news. Ginny was able to see the upside, knowing how happy it made our daughter. The following weekend, Lauren and Al came up to Boston and we all went out to dinner to celebrate.

While my wife kept her true feelings to herself, I would tell her that she was wrong about Al, especially now. I thought I was proven right. The way I looked at it at that time, Al had to be a stand-up guy. He had come back into Lauren's life when she was sick with cancer, and now he wanted to marry her, knowing full well what he was getting into. Most guys would run and hide. It's something that many times will cause a marriage to fail, so I had to take my hat off to him.

I offered to pay for the wedding, but Lauren wouldn't allow it.

"You only get one," she told me. "You got the last one. I'll handle this."

"Well, I have to do something," I said.

"If you want get the flowers, you and Mom can do that for me. How's that?"

I agreed, and went one better. I knew she had made arrangements to have the ceremony in a Catholic church in New York City not far from her apartment, with a reception to follow at Columbia University in one of their function rooms.

"Here's what else I want to do," I told her. "I'll charter a bus to shuttle the wedding party and guests attending the church service uptown to Columbia University to make things easier for everyone."

There were people coming from all over, including friends from Boston who didn't know their way around New York. Lauren thought it was a great idea, so that's what we did.

The wedding took place on an unusually balmy March day in 2006 before 150 exuberant people, including some of Lauren's doctors.

Lauren was every bit the nervous bride. She wanted everything to be perfect. She concerned herself with every detail, but more than anything she wanted to make sure that everyone was having a great time. She seemed to want to shift the focus away from herself. Joie may not have been the only one who suspected that something else was troubling the new bride, but Lauren never let on as to what that might be. At one point before the ceremony, however, Joie was alone with Lauren in a room that had a fully mirrored wall. She stopped to look at herself in her wedding dress. Her bridal gown had a low neckline, and she reached up with her finger and traced the scar on her chest. Then she looked at the beautiful bouquet of flowers she was holding and a big smile broke out across her face. She turned to Joie, still smiling.

"Does my breath smell fresh?" she asked, leaning in close to Joie.

Ginny told me later that at the start of the ceremony, she thought she experienced an anxiety attack. She didn't know how else to describe it. While I was walking Lauren down the aisle, all eyes, including Ginny's, were on the beautiful bride. A beautiful song was playing—I can't recall what it was—when Ginny suddenly broke down. She let out a soft but audible cry. She didn't understand it, but she told me that she was just afraid. Someone seated behind her touched her shoulder in support. She didn't look around to see who it was—she was too embarrassed, even though the individual probably just thought it was an emotional reaction Ginny was having to seeing her cancer-survivor daughter getting married.

At the reception, Lauren had the seating cards attached to polished red apples that symbolized both Manhattan and her health. Several of her friends had gone out to find more than one hundred of the most perfectly shaped and similar-sized red apples they could.

It may not have been the biggest wedding, but to see Lauren so happy and among all her friends, it was special.

After the reception, Al and Lauren were joined by a group of Lauren's closest friends, and they all went to a little local pub to continue the celebration into the early hours of the morning. Lauren remained in her wedding dress, and they laughed for hours. It was one great big party.

The celebration had as much to do with Lauren's hard-fought battle with lung cancer and the year and a half that it had taken from her as it was about the nuptials that brought everyone together. It is now my unqualified belief that Lauren married Al because she wanted to ease our mind and temper our concern about her. I believe she did it entirely for our security, not her own.

All of Lauren's friends felt good that she was happy and healthy and that she was starting a new life after cancer, now so simply and perfectly symbolized in a new marriage. Unfortunately, nothing was simple or perfect for Lauren anymore.

A week before the ceremony, Lauren had a call from her oncologist, who told her that something had been detected in her midsection. She was told not to worry about it at that time, but to enjoy her wedding; a week or two would not matter. They would take care of it when she returned from her honeymoon, the doctor said, adding that it was probably nothing.

But Lauren couldn't just forget it, and she considered postponing the wedding. She kept this news from her mother and me, confiding only in her closest friends, including Monica, who agreed with her this time not to tell us about the phone call from her oncologist. Monica also helped to convince Lauren to go ahead with the wedding. If it turned out to be nothing, she said, she would be disappointing a lot of people and she would have wasted precious time and energy in the planning of the event. And if it was something, she would have to deal with it whether she was married or not.

It just wasn't fair. At this stage in her life, Lauren was looking healthy again and was very happy. She was also newly married. But in the midst of these new circumstances, she was confronted with bad news. When she came back from her honeymoon she went to see her oncologist, who informed her that they had found some cancer near her right ribs. Monica and Lauren were at work when Lauren took her aside and told her that her cancer was back and that they needed to perform surgery on her right away to remove two of her ribs. Lauren was so upset that she went into the bathroom and threw up. Monica went in after her and found Lauren in tears.

"What am I going to do?" Lauren cried. "I don't want to go through this again. Why is this happening?"

Twelve

No Time for Last-Minute Commiserators

In the end, the grim reaper isn't always enshrouded in a dark hood and carrying a scythe. Sometimes, he looks like you or me, cleverly disguised in a pair of blue jeans, a Land's End twin set or a pair of sneakers.

He, or she, is a relative, or a friend, or a long-ago acquaintance who shows up, seemingly out of nowhere. Most of them are well-meaning, to be sure, but some are doing it for themselves, perhaps to make up for time lost on the front end. Whatever their motives, they're doing it on my time, precious time that I don't care to share with people who haven't been there all along.

This showing up at the end is a phenomenon a lot of so-cial workers see as people face life-threatening illnesses. "It's natural," according to Earl Collom, a social worker with the Visiting Nurse Service of New York. "People want to feel useful in any way they can, even if it's not particularly help-ful to the sick person."

One visitor arrived recently to see me at the hospital, stayed a few hours and then caught another train home. I hadn't seen her in more than two years, and while a small part of me was happy for the visit, I couldn't help but wonder where she had been all this time.

Collom said it's natural to have these feelings of resent-ment, and it's even more important to draw your own bound-ary lines. "You have to be very clear about what is working and what is not working for you. You have to tell them, 'My energy is very limited, my focus is very limited right now, so it's not a good time.'"

About three weeks ago, I got a very disturbing e-mail from a former colleague I hadn't spoken to in at least seven years. Even when we worked together we weren't particularly close. I was expecting a pleasant note.

"So-and-so tells me you are dying," the man wrote, be-fore inviting my husband and me to his farmhouse.

Now, call me crazy, but I thought the offer to be a little odd. The skeptical reporter in me questioned whether he was making the grandiose offer more for himself than for me. He

*clearly gave no thought to my reaction on the other end of
the e-mail, especially the "I hear you are dying" part.*

*My father always taught me that you honor people when
they are alive and not wait until they're dead or close to it.
I happen to agree.*

It's really all about common sense.

*When you are ill, so much is out of your control. Getting a
handle on other people's deeds—or misdeeds—is something
you can control.*

—From *Newsday*, "Life, with Cancer," May 1, 2007,
"No Time for Last-minute Commiserators,"
by Lauren Terrazzano. (This was Lauren's last installment.)

1

The following month, just before Easter, Lauren underwent
another surgery to remove the tumors, along with several ribs
where tumors were located. She got through that surgery, and again
they thought they had gotten all the cancer. Lauren had quite a lot of
pain and discomfort following the operation. Besides tissue removal,
they were excising bone, so there was more sensitivity and pain associated with the recovery. She had to go through more radiation treatments as well, though they were not as aggressive this time, and she
did not get sick, as she did before.

She had us, as always, to lean on and reassure her, but she also had
a full support system in place. Throughout her ordeal, there were
a couple of friends that she could always count on to tell it like it

was, and one of them was Leah. Lauren was never one for half-truths or sugar-coating reality, something Leah had long known about her friend. When people would tell Lauren that everything was going to be okay, Leah would often see her subtly cringe. While Lauren understood that people often uttered such platitudes out of fear or with genuine good intentions, she appreciated hearing an alternative opinion and voice. Leah became that voice. She was one of the only people who would acknowledge just how much the treatments Lauren had to undergo sucked, plain and simple.

"Sounded like you had a horrible day," Leah would say, or sometimes she would not say anything, rather than lie. Lauren found her straightforward approach refreshing. A lot of it *was* horrible, and Lauren appreciated the fact that someone knew that and could be straight with her.

During this brief period of Lauren's remission, Leah was expecting her first child. Lauren was very excited for her friend, but Leah was having a challenging pregnancy. Lauren would call her every day to see how she was doing. Leah didn't think she had any right to complain about anything to Lauren, who had gone through so much already. However, Lauren told Leah that her (Leah's) medical worries were even more significant because the life of an innocent baby was at stake. This was a point well taken by Leah, who thought that it was so like Lauren to find just the right thing to say, making Leah feel more comfortable opening up about her own discomfort and her anxieties about the health of her baby.

When Leah went into labor near the end of summer, Lauren came out to Boston to be with her. It was a wonderful time in Leah's life, and being able to share it with Lauren made it extra special. However, while visiting in the hospital with Leah and her new baby, Lauren began experiencing severe headaches. They began to be so intense that she went down to the hospital's emergency room to get checked out. Her initial fear was that the headaches might signal a brain tumor. It turned out that there was a mass behind her eye, but it was not cancerous. However, she had to endure another operation to remove the tumor.

As Lauren was recovering from this surgery at Sloan-Kettering, she got an unexpected visitor—Joe Torre, the manager of the New York Yankees, the perennial archrivals of her beloved Boston Red Sox. Lauren recognized him right away. Torre, who was a prostate cancer survivor, was at the hospital and he happened to duck into her room in order to dodge some reporters. He excused himself for intruding and explained his situation. He was very polite.

"You paid too much for Johnny Damon," Lauren said at one point, eliciting a polite laugh from the Yankee skipper.

"No one is immune from cancer," he said before he left. "It can get anyone."

2

When tumors began appearing in different parts of her body, Lauren's cancer was considered inoperable, at least as far as the recommendation of any further surgeries was concerned. The word "terminal" had not been spoken, but Lauren was running out of options. She asked her doctors what the best course of treatment should now be. They told her that the type of cancer she had was extremely aggressive and would continue to come back. Any further chemotherapy would not be effective and would only make her sick.

Her hope was fading fast when she decided to put her faith in a trial drug.

While Lauren was undergoing this experimental treatment, she decided to approach her editors about an idea she had been thinking about for several months. She wanted to chronicle her experiences of fighting and living with lung cancer in order to shed some much-needed light on a highly misunderstood disease that affected many people, and women in particular, in ways that few people realized. She got the idea after writing an article for the September 2006 issue of *Self*, a women's magazine that specializes in health, fitness, and nutrition, and related topics of health and beauty. The article Lauren contributed focused on the different stages of her treatment, starting from the time that her tumor had been discovered two years earlier. She divulged a lot of intimate feelings and emotions in her recollections of the experiences she had had at each stage of the disease and received an overwhelming response from readers (mainly women) who were thankful to her for sharing her personal story. Lauren wanted to continue what she had been doing as a journalist her entire career—tackling a taboo subject the media often failed to adequately address.

Newsday, after considering Lauren's request, quickly gave their endorsement, and Lauren immediately began working on a weekly column that would be called "Life, with Cancer."

Lauren stayed on the trial drug through October, when the first installment of her new column appeared in the paper, on Halloween day. The following week Lauren's oncologist informed her that her body was not responding to the treatment. When Lauren asked what they could try next, her doctors told her that they had done everything they could; conventional treatment had failed.

When Lauren inquired about alternative therapies they could recommend, she was advised that if there were any nontraditional medicines or treatments she wanted to try, it was up to her; but there was nothing more they could do for her at Sloan-Kettering.

3

As 2006 drew to a close, Lauren really began to take a hard look at the disease and its impact on the lives of patients and their families. From the time Lauren's first installment of "Life, with Cancer" appeared in the paper, I became aware of the impact it had on readers. Her mother and I had always been proud of her, but it was pleasing to see some of the values I tried to instill in her reflected in her writing. She didn't mince words, even when it came to an illness that was draining the life out of her; she made it clear to the readers exactly what she was experiencing.

People would stop Ginny and me all the time and tell us how much they enjoyed Lauren's "Life, with Cancer" column. Within a couple months, everyone seemed to know Lauren for this column. Sometimes complete strangers would hear our last name and make a complimentary remark about something Lauren had written in it. Some of those people had cancer themselves or knew someone who did. It was fulfilling to know that she gave those people some comfort. It truly meant a lot to hear this firsthand, and I always thanked them for sharing it with us, but it was something that would have been infinitely more satisfying if the topic of Lauren's column had been just about anything else, really.

She was telling readers around the world what her life was like living with lung cancer. It was among some of the best writing she had ever done. At the same time that she immersed herself fully in her work, just as she had before she got sick, receiving accolades and notoriety for her writing, she began to take a turn for the worse.

4

Lauren began to prepare her friends for her imminent death in different ways. She believed that it would be less devastating if she eased them into the reality of it a little at a time. How she broached the topic of her mortality with each individual was based on how much she thought the person would be able to handle.

Monica believed that Lauren thought too highly of her (Monica's) coping ability when the two of them went for a walk together in Central Park one mild winter afternoon. Monica was in the planning stages of her annual trip to Spain, and she had just asked Lauren to come along. Monica was taken by complete surprise when Lauren turned slowly to her and said, "You're going to have to get used to the idea that I'm not going to be around for long."

"Lauren, come on. Don't talk like that."

Lauren gazed at Monica with a steely cast in her eyes. Her face had almost no expression. "I'm going to die. You have to accept that. You have to get ready."

"Okay. And you have to get ready for Spain."

"No. You have to be strong now, Monica. You have to help me. You have to help my parents."

It was a sobering moment of reality for Monica, who may have been somewhat in denial after seeing Lauren come back so many times before from suffering and the brink of death with this disease.

Lauren said, "Promise me that you'll be there when I die."

It was like a blow to the gut. Monica felt as though the wind had been knocked out of her. "Of course," she stammered.

Lauren seemed to relax, given this reassurance, and they walked on.

Lauren loved and trusted her friends so much, and they loved her. I don't know what she would have done without them. They were always there for her. Ginny and I could depend on them as well. One or both of us would have been with Lauren all the time, but because of them it made it easy for Lauren to tell us to go home and not worry about her for a little while. Not that it mattered where we were, we would always worry about her, but Lauren didn't want to overburden us. On top of the trauma of witnessing her day-by-day deterioration, there was the commute back and forth to Massachusetts, her cramped apartment when we stayed over, and the expense and inconvenience of having to stay at a nearby hotel on occasion. None of these things bothered us, but Lauren was always worried about these things and it became a consideration she could exploit because she had so many good friends all living close by. I have to admit that my snoring may have had as much to do with our urged respites as anything else. Even my sleeping on the couch in the living room was keeping Lauren awake at night and preventing her from getting the rest she needed. Knowing she was in such good hands made it easier for us to leave her for a day or two.

Then Al came through and was able to get us an apartment that was owned by the *New York Times*. It was a place they kept to accommodate out-of-town guests or new employees in transition while they were looking for a permanent residence. It was located near the *New York Times* building, right in Times Square, and the newspaper was gracious enough to provide the apartment for us rent-free for as long as we needed while it was unoccupied. We would often walk the forty blocks to Lauren's apartment, but when Ginny wasn't up for it, or if the weather was bad, it was easy enough to cab it uptown.

As for how we were handling Lauren's terminal condition, it was something that we were coming to terms with in our own way. I was not so accepting. Neither of us was willing to give up on our daughter—that would never happen—but I refused to let her go without a fight, even if it was one I could never win. That's just how I am. Somewhere, there was something that could help Lauren. There had to be. I am the consummate optimist, and I always see the glass as half full, whereas my wife looks at things quite differently. Ginny didn't tell me then, but she later confided that she had known by this time that Lauren was not going to make it. My wife considers herself a realist, but I will tell her she is a pessimist. It's something we argue about from time to time, but no matter what we say, neither of us has changed, nor did it change Lauren's medical prognosis.

We spent Christmas 2006 in New York with Lauren and Al. I refused to believe it would be the last holiday we would celebrate with our daughter. We enjoyed that time together and exchanged gifts. Ginny and I gave them an American Express credit card and encouraged them to use it to take a trip somewhere. Lauren thanked us but vehemently refused to use the card, expressing her concern for our financial situation. I assured her we wouldn't have given it to them if we couldn't afford it and that we would have bought them another present of equal value that wouldn't have done her nearly as good. Finally she acquiesced, and the following week she and Al left for a brief getaway to Puerto Rico.

By early February, Lauren began to sound quite despondent in the phone conversations we had. I once again suggested that she and Al use the Amex card to go off somewhere to relax. I didn't know what in particular, if anything, might have been troubling her, but I subsequently learned that she had been arguing with Al about the alternative treatments that she had been considering and which he, apparently, did not support. Al had refused to accompany us to Houston the previous month when we went to find out more about an experimental therapy involving the use of proton beams. At that time, I was focused on finding a program that would help Lauren and keep her alive, and I did not necessarily notice everything that was going on between her and Al.

During the first week of March, Lauren had completed a new drug regimen and was recovering from the side effects when she called her mother and me to tell us she had decided to take my offer and travel south for a few days. She went to Miami. Alone.

I knew she could use the physical relief, but I was not aware of the full extent of the emotional trauma she had been experiencing. It would become clear to me later, after speaking with Lauren's friends, that the added stress Al placed on her, pitting him against me regarding the seeking of alternative cancer treatment, weighed heavily on her. Lauren returned from Florida to more bad news. Her doctors informed her that new masses had appeared on her remaining lung. A CT scan revealed three cancerous nodules, and she knew right away it was a death sentence. There was only one thing left to know, and she asked her oncologist how long she had to live. For Lauren, hearing that she would not live more than another two months was difficult enough, but it was still easier than the prospect of having to tell everyone, particularly her mother and me, which was what she had to do next.

Lauren immediately drafted a letter and e-mailed it to all of her dearest friends to give them the dire news. They responded in kind, traveling from near and far to spend time with Lauren, showing her the affection and devotion that Lauren had always extended to them.

Jessica Kowal, who had moved to Seattle in 2003, had kept in touch with Lauren all along and came to visit her in New York as soon as she got Lauren's letter.

In 2006, Tomoeh had moved to Washington, DC, with her husband and was working for the *Washington Post*. When Lauren was going through her treatments, Tomoeh would visit her in New York just about every other weekend. Then the *Post* asked Tomoeh if she would move to the New York bureau to be their Wall Street correspondent, and she jumped at it. Her husband, Archie, who was working out of the DC office for the *New York Times,* was able to transfer to his paper's office in Manhattan, so they were all together by 2007. At that time, Lauren insisted on helping the couple apartment hunt, going online and finding places for them to look at. If one was close to Lauren's own apartment, she would venture out with Tomoeh and Archie to look at the place with them and give them her advice.

Seeing Lauren only recently, Tomoeh could hardly believe that Lauren was dying. She still looked so good, and she otherwise appeared the same in every other way. She may have been ill, but she continued to concern herself with the welfare of others, especially her friends. If one of them developed a bad cold or flu, Lauren would be sure to send soup, just as she had always done.

One time, while Lauren was undergoing a chemo regimen, Dr. Ashfaq developed a cold and Lauren needed a soup courier. She asked Tomoeh to stop by a particular deli on the Upper West Side to pick up some chicken soup and deliver it to Dr. Ashfaq at North Shore Medical Hospital, which she did. Lauren would have brought it herself if she hadn't been in treatment and so susceptible to germs. Tomoeh did it gladly, even though she did not know Dr. Ashfaq at the time. Her friends began to tell her they were okay, even if they were sick, so that Lauren wouldn't worry about them while she was very ill herself.

Before the end of March, Lauren had called Leah's mother and father so they could break the news to Leah. Lauren thought it would soften the blow a little for Leah if it came from her parents first. It did not. When Lauren was able to tell Leah herself about her terminal status, neither of them could control their emotions. Leah flew out to New York the next week to see her friend. It was March 26, two days before Lauren's birthday. The celebration was subdued, with only her closest friends and family around her. By then, the process had already begun to accelerate and it had taken a savage toll on Lauren physically and emotionally.

On April 1, Lauren made it official, seemingly accepting her fate when she drafted another letter that she sent by e-mail to all her friends. It was her way of saying good-bye and thanking them for their love and friendship. Ginny and I didn't know anything about the letter at the time. She wrote:

> i'm sorry i have been out of touch. we have shut the phone off, the ringer, the machine. i was released friday but have been in tremendous pain. my abdomen is still swollen with fluid, and that puts pressure on my diaphragm, which puts pressure in my one remaining lung, which makes it very difficult to breathe. so I am having a tough time. my parents are here with me and we are taking it moment by moment. thank you for all your wonderful birthday cards and gifts and for your prayers. i am trying to hang in there but it is very hard. everything seems to be failing. We are looking into hospice alternatives. Please say a prayer but I think my miracle days are over. I will try to be in touch, but if i am not, please know how much your friendship means to me and that I know how loved i have been over the past several years. I will take that with me. And please keep this e-mail among us.

> —LT

5

E den Laikin was raised Jewish, but she only practiced her religion on the High Holy Days. She was more a spiritual than a religious person, and that was part of the relationship that she had with Lauren. She could talk with Lauren about subjects like death in a way that no one else could.

About two years before Lauren got sick, a good friend of Eden's named Brian, who had survived AIDS as well as the trauma of being sexually abused by a priest when he was a child, was dying from liver cancer. Before he passed, Eden got very close to Brian, and in the process she learned about forgiveness and grace and the need that terminal people have to talk with someone about death and faith. One day, when he was near the end, Brian told Eden that he needed to speak with someone about it but he didn't trust the church. He asked Eden if she thought she could handle it. Eden said she could, and although it wasn't easy, it comforted Brian to express his fears and thoughts on the subject. Eden stayed up with him talking, until just hours before he died. It was an experience she would not soon forget. Lauren later helped her write his obituary for *Newsday*.

Eden had been formally trained in Reiki, a Japanese spiritual practice that uses a technique commonly called palm healing as a form of complementary therapy. Its practitioners believe that they are transferring universal energy through the palms, which allows for self-healing and a state of equilibrium. It is also believed to help ease the transition from this life to the next.

Earlier in the year that Lauren was diagnosed with lung cancer,

Eden's sister-in-law Joanne was diagnosed with ovarian cancer. Eden spent a lot of time with her, taking her to chemo treatments and doctor's appointments and doing Reiki on her when she had pain.

Being so close to Brian and Joanne in their last hours helped Eden prepare for Lauren's treatment. Eden administered Reiki to Lauren where she had pain, or whenever Lauren became overly anxious or stressed. The treatment always seemed to calm her down. When Lauren began writing her weekly column from home because it became too much for her to travel to *Newsday*'s Melville office, Eden would sometimes join her and they would work together in her living room. The editors were very flexible in that regard, granting a number of other reporters the same privilege so there would always be someone with Lauren, whether it was to take her to her treatments or just to spend time with her.

Sometimes Lauren would open up to Eden and they would talk about their beliefs and about life. One time, Lauren started to cry and said, "I don't want to die."

It may have been the first time Lauren, used that word in Eden's presence. "I know you don't, babe," Eden told her. "What is supposed to happen will happen regardless of what doctors and tests say. Live in the day, in the moment, that's all any of us have. This moment. Look where your feet are. In this moment, you're okay."

Eden knew that she was the only one Lauren would freely talk with about dying. Eden had been prepared.

One night, over dinner at Lauren's favorite Italian restaurant, near her apartment, she asked, "Eeds, what do you think happens when we die? Do you believe in heaven?"

Tomoeh, who was with them at the time, was shocked by the bluntness of Lauren's question.

"Yes," Eden said. "I believe there is a heaven, and after we pass there is no more pain or sickness or worry or any negativity, just peace. I believe we can still communicate from this side to the other side. And no matter how things appear now or how you feel, God loves you."

Eden believed this comforted Lauren, and I believed it did, as well. I had no problems with Lauren seeking spiritual or physical comfort by any means.

I was still not ready to give up on her. As Lauren's future fell further in doubt, I accelerated my efforts of finding a miracle cure, researching everything I could find on the subject of alternative cancer treatments in the current medical journals. One I thought to be very promising was close to being approved for human trials. Researchers at the University of Alberta, Edmonton, Canada, had shown that dichloroacetate (DCA), an "off-patent" drug that was odorless, colorless, inexpensive, and relatively nontoxic, caused regression in several cancers, including lung, breast, and brain tumors. I wrote a letter to the head of the DCA research team and requested more information on the drug. I shared all my findings with Al as well as Lauren.

One morning in early April, Lauren called me and asked me to back off making any further treatment suggestions to Al. Apparently my zeal to find a way to halt the progression of my daughter's lung cancer had become a frustration to him. Much to my dismay, Lauren asked me to cease and desist sending Al any further e-mails or placing any calls to him regarding the subject. She just wanted to keep the peace, but I would soon discover that she and Al had been fighting about money all along.

6

As Lauren's vital signs dropped dangerously low, she became very weak. She was only given medication to help her tolerate the pain. She was in and out of the hospital for a while, until finally she was unable to leave. There, she was never alone in her fifteenth-floor private room, number 1501, at Memorial Sloan-Kettering Cancer Center. Her mother and I were always there, along with any number of Lauren's friends. Among them was Leah, who saw her childhood friend dying before her eyes. As difficult as that was, Leah could also see how much it hurt Lauren to watch the trauma that her mother and I had to endure, and that made it all the more distressing for everyone

Nearer to the end, Lauren sometimes misdirected her anger and frustration about the loss she felt she was saddling us with. She knew her death would devastate us, and her mounting guilt about leaving us alone reached a level where she would suddenly lash out or say things that may have seemed harsh.

"I told them to adopt," she once snapped at Leah. "Why didn't they listen to me?"

Leah was aware that Lauren had never liked being an only child, but they both realized that she probably would not have turned out to be the person she was if she had had a sibling. She had to learn to blaze her own trail in life, and that helped her develop her strong, independent spirit.

Lauren talked a lot to Leah about Ginny and me at this time. "What's going to happen to them?" she would ask over and over again.

When Lauren's kidneys and liver began shutting down, there were discussions about putting her into a hospice facility. Her abdomen swelled and she became bedridden. A drain had to be inserted into her stomach to keep the fluid from building up.

The night Leah stayed overnight in her room at the hospital, Lauren had a craving for ziti with mozzarella cheese, even though she could hardly eat. It had been a while since she could eat anything besides soup. Leah got the ziti for her and they ate together, even though Lauren only had a couple of bites. It was nice, because they had always enjoyed dining together. They had an Italian meal together like they used to, and Leah got to say good-bye in person.

The last few days, Lauren was in and out of consciousness, but she awoke suddenly one afternoon, lucid and seemingly strong, and called Leah. They had a real conversation, not talking about her illness or death or anything like that. They just talked as friends. Lauren did tell Leah that she had been given a great gift. Leah knew what she meant. Lauren was telling her friend to appreciate every day of her life.

I called Leah when her doctors said that Lauren had twenty-four hours left before the disease she fought so hard against for nearly three years claimed her life. I had a sense of relief, as well as overwhelming grief, which Leah undoubtedly heard in my voice when I told her the news. There was much suffering for everyone in those final days.

Unbeknownst to Ginny and me, Al and his father began looking into finding hospice care for Lauren, with apparent plans to move her from Sloan-Kettering into one of these facilities to die. They had one all picked out when they called to invite Ginny and I to visit the facility on May 8. It was Calvary Hospital in the Bronx, and it was quite nice, actually.

While part of me understood why he had been searching for these final accommodations, the invitation took me by complete surprise. I could only wonder if Sloan-Kettering was recommending it or if they were otherwise booting us out for some reason. It didn't seem to make a whole lot of sense, especially considering the top-of-the-line care that Lauren was receiving right where she was. It felt like we were being roped into this, and more significantly, so was Lauren, who Al was making plans for without consulting.

I would very soon come to realize why he began looking in that direction.

7

On Thursday, May 10, Monica was at the hospital all day with us. There were many other visitors that day, and Lauren was quite active. She seemed happy, and she smiled a lot. When she expressed a craving for Spanish food, I ran out to get takeout. Lauren was also paid a visit by the hospital chaplain, who came in to administer Last Rites to her. On Friday, Monica spent the day at Lauren's bedside with Ginny and me, none of us knowing what to expect that day. It was a much quieter day and Lauren was less active. She didn't speak much and she slept fitfully, but she rested comfortably.

Saturday presented a different set of challenges that none of us could have expected. It was about 8:30 that morning when I took a phone call from Al. He stated that he was in Lauren's hospital room and announced that Lauren wanted to speak with me. In the next instant I heard my daughter's barely coherent voice on the other end.

"Daddy," she pleaded, "you have to help Al pay for the private room charges."

Listening to her struggling to speak through the heavy pain medication she was taking, I had barely heard the words she said.

Once I comprehended the request, and although it wasn't an appropriate topic of discussion at that time or something I felt Lauren should be concerned about, my initial reaction was to offer whatever help I could.

"Of course, sweetheart," I told her. "Don't you worry. I'll take care of it."

"Thank you, Daddy."

Before I could say anything else, Al was back on the line.

"Frank," he began, "the hospital is requesting payment. When you get to the hospital today, could you go to billing and pay for Lauren's private room charges?"

He told me that the charges had been accruing since May 1, and at $600 a day the total had surpassed $7,000. He also made mention that he had gotten us the *New York Times* corporate apartment we had been staying in rent-free; I felt he was implying that because of this wonderful gesture by his employers, we were obligated to pay the extra room charges. "Okay?" he concluded.

I was taken aback by all this. It was an unusual request, the timing was poor, and it was needlessly upsetting Lauren, but I remained inclined to do whatever was needed.

I asked Al about his current financial situation and told him that I intended to take an equity loan out against our home to ensure that there were enough funds to help with any future expenses associated with Lauren's medical care.

Yes, I was still thinking ahead.

Al's response to me was, "That is not your concern right now. Just pay the hospital. Okay?"

The call ended.

The more I thought about the exchange I had with Al, the more it bothered me, particularly how he purposefully threw the *Times* apartment up in my face.

Irate, I turned to Ginny and said, "I think you were right about him."

I then contacted Lauren's friends Tomoeh and Archie Tse. Archie, a graphic artist for the *New York Times*, and they were temporarily residing in the same apartment complex as Ginny and I. I told them about the conversation I had with Al, and I was so infuriated by then that I was resolved to contact the newspaper, thank them for their hospitality, and let them know that we would be vacating the apartment on Monday.

"We'll try to find a sublet or get a room at a local hotel," I told them.

Tomoeh and Archie pleaded with me not to leave. They even offered their apartment for our use, volunteering to temporarily move out and stay with friends. This truly generous gesture by terrific friends of Lauren caused me to reconsider my hasty decision.

When Ginny and I arrived at the hospital, Tomoeh and Archie were already there, but Al was not. He didn't come back the rest of the day.

Lauren slept most of the day, but upon waking she asked for Monica, who came by that evening and announced that she was going to stay the night.

"You guys need a break," she told us. "Get some rest tonight."

Monica got Lauren to eat a little, and for dessert she had some Italian ice that Monica had brought with her. Lauren found the flavored slush very refreshing. She usually didn't have an appetite for much else.

Dr. Flores came in at one point and Lauren talked with him briefly. She asked him to make sure she did not suffer. She told Monica that she was not so afraid of death, but fearful of how it would happen, dreading suffocation and not being able to breathe. The doctor assured her that would not happen, that she would not feel any pain or anxiety. When he left, Lauren asked Monica if she should believe him.

"He's never lied to you before," Monica said.

Lauren then asked Monica to be sure she did not suffer.

Monica told her not to worry. "I promise," Monica said. "I'll be right here with you the entire time." And she was. Ginny and I left late and returned early the next morning.

Sunday, May 13, was Mother's Day. Monica reported that Lauren had slept through the night. Lauren was completely out of it when several doctors came in and examined her. They determined that her organs were failing fast and we knew she did not have much time left. When Lauren noticed us she perked up a little. Mother and daughter embraced, and Lauren whispered "Happy Mother's Day, Mom," and everyone had tears in their eyes.

Monica said she was going to see her own mother. Lauren seemed happy about that and asked Monica to say hello to her mom for her.

It had been a long weekend for Monica, who was afraid that Lauren was going to die and that she wouldn't be there as she had promised she would be. But Lauren was tired, and as soon as Monica left she fell asleep. She didn't wake up until around 6:00 that evening, and the first person she asked for was Monica. Al was a no-show that day, but Tomoeh, who had since joined us, called Monica on her cell phone. She picked up right away.

"Hi, Tomoeh," Monica said. "Everything all right?"

"Hi, Monica. Yes. I'm at the hospital. Lauren's been asking for you. She wants to talk to you."

"Great. Put her on."

Tomeoh placed her phone gently against Lauren's ear.

"Monica?" Lauren said weakly.

"Hi, Lauren?" Monica asked. "Did you have anything to eat today?"

"A little," Lauren said. "I'm calling to wish your mother a Happy Mother's Day."

"That's so sweet of you. Thank you. I'll be sure to tell her. I promise. Do you want me to come over tonight, Lauren?"

"No," Lauren said. "We'll see each other tomorrow."

"Okay. I'll be there early."

"Goodnight, babe."

"Goodnight."

Ginny and I stayed over in the room with Lauren that night. Sleep was all but impossible, but we wanted to be there.

8

By the next morning, Ginny needed to go back to the apartment to get some rest. It was Monday, May 14, and I stayed at the hospital with my daughter and was grateful that I got to spend a little bit of time alone with her on my sixty-sixth birthday. What turned out to be our final moments together as father and daughter, spent mostly in quiet reflection, was intruded upon when Al walked into the room. After not seeing or speaking to me for two days, the first words out of his mouth were to inform me of his decision to move Lauren into Calvary Hospital because she was not receiving adequate care at Sloan-Kettering. He never asked about Lauren, how she was doing, or what her doctors were saying.

I immediately challenged him, insisting that we had all witnessed the excellent care that Lauren—and all of us—had benefited from during the time we had been there. I barked that he had not been around the past two days to observe the kind and considerate treatment we had been shown by the doctors, nurses, and the entire hospital staff as Lauren lay near death.

I was getting hot, and he backed down on moving Lauren out to Calvary Hospital. He still did not inquire about Lauren, but moved on to what was really on his mind.

"Did you pay the private room charges?" he asked me.

"No," I said. "And I'm not going to, either."

"You're not going to honor your daughter's last wishes?"

I could not believe what I was hearing. Given the circumstances, I don't know that I've ever heard anything so disrespectful, callous, and selfish in all my life.

"You're an asshole," I said in a fit of rage as I lunged at him.

If the door hadn't opened at that exact moment, and if it had been anyone other than Dr. Flores entering the room, I'm certain we would have come to blows right there in Lauren's $600-a-day private room as she slept through the final hours of her life.

Al excused himself and stepped out of the room after Dr. Flores greeted everyone. Then the doctor walked over to Lauren's bed and spoke softly to her. She responded to his voice and her eyes opened slightly. She smiled a little when she saw him. "Remember what you promised me?" she said faintly.

"Don't worry," Dr. Flores said. "I'm here." He kept his promise, and he spent much of the day coming in to check on Lauren.

"Is this it?" I mustered up the strength to ask him at one point.

He nodded solemnly.

I called Monica first to tell her that Lauren was not doing well and that she should get to the hospital as soon as she could. She picked up Ginny on the way, and when they arrived Lauren was making a rasping sound in her throat, as if she was having difficulty breathing. Lauren drifted in and out of consciousness and seemed to be experiencing hallucinations. At one point she woke up and said, "What are you all doing around me?" That seemed to really freak Monica out.

Several times, we all thought Lauren had died as her breathing seemed to stop, but she always came back. It had been a long and stressful several days for everyone, and by that night we all needed to rest. But we did not want Lauren to pass while we were asleep. I stayed in the hospital room that night with my dying daughter while Monica drove Ginny back to our courtesy apartment in Times Square.

The following morning, Tuesday, May 15, Lauren's doctors told me that she would pass away that day. I quickly phoned Monica and together we contacted everyone we could to tell them what was happening. We were all waiting for the end to come. To everyone's surprise, though, Lauren woke up and spoke a little. She asked for ice cream, though she was struggling to breathe. Nurses kept coming in to adjust her oxygen levels, but Dr. Flores thought that this was needlessly prolonging the inevitable and keeping her alive artificially, something Lauren did not want. He suggested having her ventilator turned off, and we all agreed, though it was a painful decision. He continued to administer sedatives to her so that she was not in any pain.

Waiting for Lauren to pass away was the most difficult couple of hours for us and for everyone in the room to endure. Despite Dr. Flores's reassurances, Lauren appeared to be suffering, talking incoherently, and after a while it was so tormenting that I started thinking, *Please, God, just take her.*

Eden did Reiki on Lauren as she took her last breaths.

"It's okay, Lauren," Eden said. "You don't have to fight anymore."

Eden felt as if Lauren was finally ready. Lauren, who continued to worry about us right until the end, had demonstrated this once more by refusing to die on Mother's Day two days before, or on the following day, my birthday.

At 11:45 PM on May 15, Monica and her partner Veronica, Eden, Al, Karla Schuster, Tomoeh and Archie, as well as Dr. Flores, were all in Lauren's room with Ginny and me as Lauren took her last breaths. Monica's sister had abruptly excused herself moments before. Despite the fact that she was a nurse and had seen many people pass away, she was unable to stay in the room to see Lauren die. Everyone was watching Lauren when she suddenly moved her head slightly from one side to the other and took a long, deep breath. There was a rattling noise in her throat, a final exhalation, and she was gone. Life seemed to leave her face when her last breath left her body. All at once her skin took on the look of pure porcelain.

We all wept as we said our final good-byes. The overwhelming sadness was nearly countermanded by a dread sense of relief that Lauren's agony was finally over, and that, in a sense, ours was, too.

After the hospital attendants came in and removed Lauren from the room in our presence, we remained there for a moment without her. None of us knew what to do, and I realized that this was how it was going to be for a while. We embraced one another, and then I supported Ginny as we all made our way out of the room together.

9

Lauren's funeral services were held in New York at the Frank E. Campbell Funeral Home on Madison Avenue and 81st Street in

Manhattan. In 1994, the large and elegant mortuary buried Jackie Onassis, who Lauren, like so many people, greatly admired as a women of elegance and strength. Because of Jackie O., Lauren told her closest friends that she wanted to have her wake at Campbell's as well. Lauren had made all of the arrangements herself months in advance so that her mother and I would not have to do any of it. She even chose the image on the front of the prayer card. It was far from conventional. Instead of one of the multitude of saints and martyrs or other traditional religious depictions, the black and white photo featured a picture of a bunch of people careening down a roller coaster, arms raised, screaming and laughing and having fun. For the back of her prayer card, Lauren selected a portion of Seamus Heaney's poem, "Clearances," written in memory of his mother. She had chosen photos of herself for the albums that were placed around the funeral parlor. She didn't want to burden us with any of those details. She had even specifically asked Joe Haberstroh of *Newsday* to write her obituary for the paper.

Thursday, May 17, was the first of two consecutive nights of Lauren's wake. What I thought would be a positively unbearable experience of having to endure such a protracted session of grief in public turned out to be an enlightening one for both Ginny and me. We were honored to meet so many of Lauren's friends and colleagues and students who came to pay their respects and offer kind words of consolation to us. The multitude of tributes was overwhelming.

The second evening was attended primarily by family members and close friends from the Boston area.

Lauren had arranged to have the funeral Mass in the same church that she had been married in barely a year earlier. The funeral home provided a limousine to take us from our apartment to their chapel for a brief last visitation with Lauren before proceeding to the church for the 10:00 AM service.

Despite everything I had been through with Lauren's terminal illness, nothing could have prepared me for this day. For me, the reality that my daughter was really gone hit home at the church service.

While I may not have been a devout Catholic, I was taught that God was compassionate and that he gave his only son to be sacrificed so that others might benefit and reach the kingdom of heaven. I like to think that Lauren is now in a place like that, but I have had a difficult time forgiving God for taking Lauren at such a young age. There is some consolation in the knowledge that Lauren did so much good during her short life, helping many people, especially children and the elderly.

In looking around church that day, I saw the pews full of Lauren's coworkers, colleagues, and friends from all over the world. In the rear was a modest group of homeless men and women who appeared to be taking shelter inside the church; a few appeared to be sleeping, others listened intermittently to the eulogies, but upon closer inspection I saw that they were sitting in quiet reverence, mourning the loss of a person who had been among the more ardent advocates of their plight.

One of the people she had asked to speak at her funeral was Sylvia, whom Lauren hoped would relate some of the more lighthearted stories and good times they shared. In her remembrance, Sylvia mentioned how Lauren liked to give funny little nicknames to everyone, and how she would make them up for strangers and acquaintances alike. She talked about how much Lauren enjoyed laughing and never held back even in places where it was less than appropriate. She brought up the time the two of them were in one of the little cubicles at the hospital while Lauren was getting her chemotherapy treatment and they started laughing out of control about something and could not stop.

"Everyone was looking at us like we were crazy," she said, "and we almost got kicked out of the hospital. I can't remember what we were laughing so hard about, but it was probably over a funny name we had given to one of the doctors or nurses."

Dina, who had traveled from Guatemala, thought it was nice that she and all of Lauren's friends were together again, celebrating their friend's life just as they had done at her wedding the year before. She remembered how the bridesmaids, and all the girls, really, had done the usual prewedding drill, including getting facials at a fancy spa by a woman with a thick Russian accent, and mani-pedis at an Upper West Side Vietnamese salon. They got to spend all that time together—talking, getting to know each other—all of them so different, from different places and different times in Lauren's life, but all sharing that moment with Lauren. It was a very emotional wedding, and fourteen months later they were all back together, not only to say their good-byes to Lauren, but to share how each of them knew her and to keep her memory alive.

Fourteen months earlier, Lauren had told each of them what they meant to her in private, personal conversations. Dina recalled the night before Lauren's wedding in 2006, Dina sitting beside her friend in her darkened apartment, when Lauren slowly turned to her and expressed a heartfelt thank-you for her enduring friendship.

The day after Lauren's funeral, in the cab ride to the airport, Dina thought about that night and cried like a baby.

10

Lauren was cremated, as per her wishes, and we stayed in New York until her ashes were ready. On May 22, I collected half of my daughter's remains (Al receiving the other half) from the funeral home and informed Lauren's close and faithful friends of our decision to return to our home in Massachusetts the following morning, which we did.

For those who could not make it to New York, we had a church service for Lauren in Hull, Massachusetts. The Greers were among the attendees. Katy gave Ginny and me a big hug and offered her condolences, then she told us a story that touched us both. Katy said that an aunt had given her a toy stuffed tiger when she was young, and Lauren had always admired it. Lauren would ask Katy all the time if she could have it, but as a child Katy was not willing to part with it. She kept it into adulthood, and when she first learned that Lauren was sick she immediately shipped the tiger to New York as a symbol of their friendship. Despite the passage of time, the repairs, and popped seams, the stuffed animal had survived, just like their friendship.

I remember seeing the tiger in Lauren's bedroom on the pillow. I had wondered where it came from, and now I knew. There was a story behind everything and everyone that Lauren touched, and this was one more thing I discovered about my daughter that I had not known before.

How things had changed since that fateful day in September 2004. For Ginny and me, our home was changed forever. An aura of sadness settled like a dust layer over everything. It was like living in a museum. Everything reminded Ginny and me of our daughter: the end table and the lamp, the living room furniture—given to us by Lauren as housewarming gifts when we had moved into our new home; the photographs of Lauren around the house; a few of the many awards she received for her work as a journalist.

Today, another table in the room displays the urn containing Lauren's ashes, and it is surrounded by many more photos of Lauren and her closest friends in happier times.

But the most beautiful and most symbolic representation of Lauren is the rosebush in front of our house that flowers abundantly every year, sometimes up until Christmas. Lauren had purchased the rosebush for us before she had gotten sick, rescuing it from the discount rack at Home Depot. The plant was in pretty dire shape, and no one thought it was going to make it except for Lauren. We didn't even want to plant it, but Lauren insisted, and it has flourished ever since.

We continue to use the beautiful blooms from the rosebush that Lauren resurrected. They adorn our dinner table for guests and keep the memory of our daughter alive.

All this time later, Lauren's friends also continue to be there for us, checking in on us, letting us know that they are thinking about us and remembering Lauren. It is of great comfort to hear from them, especially on Lauren's birthday and on May 15. The memorial kite runs I make on those days remain the deepest connection I have to my daughter. It will be something I will do until I'm physically unable to do so! As I complete this book, we have just marked the fifth year since Lauren's passing. She has been gone longer now than she had lived with the disease, and lung cancer continues to claim lives every day all around the world. However, there is a certain measure of comfort in knowing that Lauren will continue to help people, giving them hope and comfort through this telling of her life story. I believe she would have liked that.

This was confirmed to me during Lauren's last birthday kite run on March 28, 2012.

Ginny was unable to accompany me, but I was not alone on the beach that day. There was a man walking toward me, and when we converged near the edge of the shore we struck up a conversation. He asked me about the kite and I told him all about Lauren. He proceeded to tell me about his life, which was almost destroyed by an addiction to drugs, which he has since beaten. He is now clean and healthy, and in talking with him I thought of Lauren. This man's story is one Lauren would have wanted to hear and write about. That he had turned his life around and was now in a position to help others by relating his experiences was something I *know* Lauren would have liked.

THE END

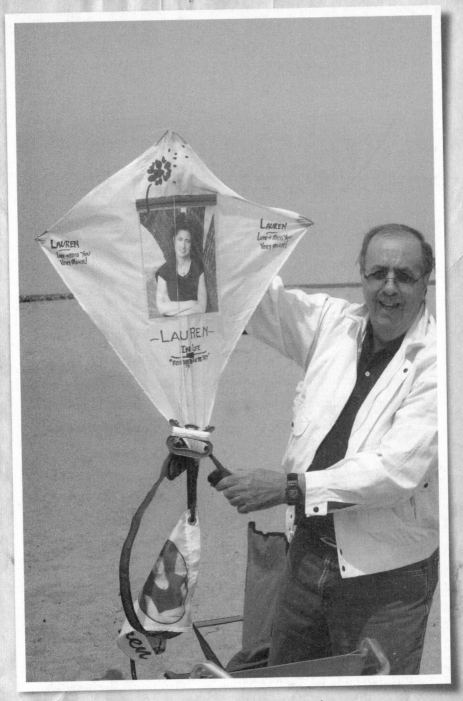

Lauren's father holding her memorial kites, which is flown on the anniversaries of her birth and her passing.
© Frank Terrazzano

About the Authors

Frank Terrazzano is a native of Boston. He worked for more than thirty years in the frozen-food industry and was responsible for purchasing as well as production planning and scheduling for Louise's Home Style Ravioli, the largest manufacturer of Italian pasta products in New England. Among his hobbies that include gardening and cooking, he shared a passion for photography and kite flying with his daughter, Lauren. He and his wife Virginia (Ginny) have been married since November 8, 1964. They reside in southeastern Massachusetts. Lauren was their only child.

Paul Lonardo is a talented writer and a publicity dynamo, which has helped to drive strong media attention to his previous book, *Caught in the Act.* His books include *Thrill Killers: A True Story of Innocence and Murder Without Conscience,* a collaboration with the lead detective who investigated the double homicide chronicled in the book and *From the Ashes: Surviving the Station Nightclub Fire,* coauthored with Gina Russo, a survivor of the 2003 nightclub fire in Rhode Island that killed one hundred people. Paul attended Columbia College, a film school in Hollywood, California, and studied screenwriting. He received a BA in English from the University of Rhode Island.